The Big Book of EVEN MORE
Therapeutic Activity Ideas
for Children and Teens

The Big Book of EVEN MORE Therapeutic Activity Ideas for Children and Teens

Inspiring Arts-Based Activities and Character Education Curricula

Lindsey Joiner

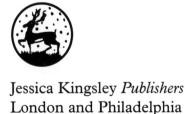

Jessica Kingsley *Publishers*
London and Philadelphia

First published in 2016
by Jessica Kingsley Publishers
73 Collier Street
London N1 9BE, UK
and
400 Market Street, Suite 400
Philadelphia, PA 19106, USA

www.jkp.com

Library of Congress Cataloging in Publication Data
A CIP catalog record for this book is available from the Library of Congress

British Library Cataloguing in Publication Data
A CIP catalogue record for this book is available from the British Library

ISBN 978 1 84905 749 3
eISBN 978 1 78450 196 9

Printed and bound in Great Britain

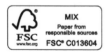

To EGJ

May these words of my mouth and this meditation of my heart be pleasing in your sight, LORD, my Rock and my Redeemer.

Psalm 19:14, Holy Bible, New International Version®

Contents

Chapter 4: Month-by-Month Character Education Activities 137

Chapter 5: Bibliotherapy Activities 208

Chapter 6: Hands-On Activities 236

Introduction

It is hard to believe that it has been almost five years since my first book (*The Big Book of Therapeutic Activities for Children and Teens: Inspiring Arts-Based Activities and Character Education Curricula*) was published. Life has brought quite a few changes for me since that time, including a change of position from a community mental health agency to a school setting, and the birth of my two children. As with any major life and career changes, I have had to adapt the things I do for a new setting and population. In a community mental health center, I had more time to complete longer projects and spent more time working with groups. In the school setting as well as in other experiences I have had since the publication of my first book, time tends to be more limited and often my work is with individuals. As a result, I have had to create new activities that work with individuals and can be completed in brief amounts of time. This book includes many of these activities that I have developed in my practice as a counselor and behavior specialist since the publication of my first book.

Even though I have experienced a lot of change over the past few years, I continue to be a strong supporter of the use of creativity and expressive arts activities in counseling and related programming with children and teens. The children and teens I work with are actively engaged in the counseling process as a result of these activities. I have observed tremendous growth in the areas of social skills, conflict resolution, anger management skills, and positive thinking with the children and teens with whom I work that I do not believe would be possible without the use of art-based activities as a means to teach these therapeutic concepts.

While this book offers similar creative and fun activities and projects to my first book, there are some differences. Many of the activities in this book can be used with individuals or adapted for application with a group. While some of the activities require more time than others, most can be completed within 30 minutes. Some of the activities work well with young children and other activities are more appropriate for preteens and teens, but many can be adapted for either population. Most of the materials needed are readily available and inexpensive. Many times they are common household or office items that you may already have available to you. There are handouts or templates that accompany many of the activities to make it easy for the user to copy and quickly begin the activity. There are ideas for adapting the activities to different populations and settings. Please feel free to modify any activity to make it work for the individual or group in your situation.

Each of the activities is presented in the same format. The purpose (or goal) of the activity is listed first. Next, the materials needed to complete the activity or project are listed. A description of the activity is included with detailed instructions for its completion. Every activity also includes a section with variations of the activity that gives additional ideas for how to use the activity, how to adapt it, or how to display the completed activities or projects. Finally, there is a section with discussion questions to help facilitate the session and encourage communication with the participants throughout the activity. Any necessary handouts or templates are also included and are ready for reproduction.

The book is organized into six chapters. The first chapter includes icebreaker activities. These are activities that can be quickly completed (usually in ten minutes or less). The icebreaker activities help to open the session in a non-threatening way. The activities in this chapter also help to build rapport and a relationship with the participant or group. I often complete the icebreaker activity along with the participant, which seems to put the participant at ease with the process. The next chapter in the book is called Shape It Up Series (Activities Using Shapes) and includes a variety of activities that teach therapeutic and character education topics using shapes. Many include handouts or templates that just need to be copied and are ready to use with the participant. There are activities in this section that would be appropriate for participants of all ages. Most of the activities in this section can be used in work with groups or individuals. The third chapter of the book includes visual and expressive arts activities. There are several activities in this section that include the use of collage, drawing, painting, writing, and other methods to teach, discuss, and encourage the development of a variety of therapeutic skills, including positive thinking, coping skills, anger management skills, following directions, communication skills, healthy self-expression, and social skills. Many of the activities in this section can be adapted for group or individual sessions. While some require an extended block of time, most can be completed within 20 to 30 minutes or broken down into steps to complete over several sessions. This section includes activities that would work with a wide variety of ages and populations. The fourth chapter includes ideas for monthly character education activities. There are two activities per month, which coordinate with holidays, seasons, or other significant events associated with the month. The activities teach a character education concept or a therapeutic lesson through expressive arts activities or other creative projects. Many of these activities make great displays for bulletin boards or other school spaces. If your setting has a positive behavior support program in place, many of these activities could be easily incorporated in this program. The activities in this setting can be easily adapted for different ages, populations, and settings. The fifth chapter features bibliotherapy activities, which use popular children's books to teach character education concepts and therapeutic lessons. Each lesson includes extension activities to reinforce the concept presented in the book. Most of the activities in this section would be appropriate for elementary aged participants. The final chapter includes activities for teaching therapeutic concepts through the completion of hands-on activities and experiments. These activities are fun for participants of all ages.

As a counselor and behavior specialist, I have learned the importance of organization, consistency, and routine when working with children and teens. It helps to be prepared for the session ahead of time, with all the materials needed already organized and ready to use. Utilizing a consistent and structured schedule for sessions helps children and teens know what to expect and learn the behavioral expectations and routine. Some children and teens may be initially resistant to completing some of the activities. While a full discussion of resistance is beyond the scope of this book, a few suggestions are noted below. Remind participants that there is no right or wrong way to complete any of the activities in this book. They will not be judged or graded on the final product, it is the process that is important. Do not force the participants to share their artwork or put them "on the spot," but instead give them the time and space to create. As they become more comfortable with the process, discussion and sharing about the activity will become easier. I often complete activities along with the participants to develop rapport with them and help put them at ease. I have found that when participants observe me completing the activity and see that I am willing to do what I ask them to do, they generally become more willing to participate themselves. Give the participants choice and options when they are completing the activity. Try not to correct if they are not completing the activity exactly as it is designed. By observing the individuals, you may learn a new and unique way to complete the activity. Remember, there is no "one size fits all" approach. Adapt the activities to the needs of the participants.

When working with groups, the use of a basic behavior plan may also help with encouraging the group members to participate and display a good attitude. From the beginning, set ground rules with the group and be sure that all participants understand the expectations and purpose of the activity. Consider developing a points system so that group members may earn points for participating and attempting to complete the activity, displaying positive social skills, and exhibiting a good attitude during the group time. The points that each group member earns can be exchanged for a special snack, a reward, or time to engage in a preferred activity at the end of session. As the group members become more and more willing to participate, the rewards can be faded out. If everyone is willing to participate except one group member, proceed with the rest of the group. Praise the positive behaviors of the group members who are participating while trying to make the activity as fun and engaging as possible. The group member may become more willing to participate when he or she sees all of the other children having fun and receiving praise. Try to stay calm and positive no matter what the situation.

Confidentiality is a critical issue for groups. It is important that confidentiality of information is discussed within the group in an age-appropriate way before beginning the group sessions. Do this as part of an informed consent process, which should include a discussion of group rules, expectations, confidentiality, and the limits of confidentiality. While it should be emphasized that all information discussed in the group should remain confidential, the group leader should let the group members know that confidentiality cannot be guaranteed within a group setting. Confidentiality should be frequently reviewed and group members should be reminded of the importance of creating a safe place to share with others. Be sure to pay attention to any conflicts or tension in the group and address these in an open and honest manner as soon as they arise so that the unity and trust with the group are not impacted.

At times, some of the activities and projects may bring up difficult emotions or memories for participants. Group leaders will have to use their best judgment to decide how to address the issue. For some concerns that come up, the group leader and other members may be able to offer valuable feedback, insight, and suggestions for how to deal with the issue. However, there are other issues that may arise within the group setting that may not be appropriate for discussion and feedback within the group. Examples might include abuse, neglect, trauma, and related issues. The group leader may need to discuss these issues in private with the individual depending on the nature of the issues, the maturity level of the group, the setting, and other factors. The group leader will need to communicate with the participant's parent or guardian and consider a referral to more intensive counseling or therapeutic services. Always consult with a colleague as well as the ethical guidelines for your profession if you are unsure how to handle a difficult situation within your practice.

The ideas in this book are a collection of activities that I have developed and adapted as part of my practice as a counselor and behavior specialist working with children and teens. These activities have been instrumental in helping me relate to the children and teens with whom I work. Not only have the activities helped the children and teens learn and implement new skills in areas such as social skills, positive thinking, coping skills, anger management, and conflict resolution, but the use of the creative activities within this book has made the process enjoyable for them as well. It is my hope that you and the children and teens you work with will have the same experience with the activities and projects provided in this book. Thank you for selecting this book and best wishes in your practice of the activities.

CHAPTER 1

Icebreakers

STATUS UPDATE

Materials needed

- Copies of the Status Update Handout
- Markers/pens

Purpose of the activity

- To put individuals at ease and build rapport for the session
- To express thoughts and feelings about current events and situations
- To provide insight into the individuals' thoughts and feelings

Description of the activity

Explain to the individuals that just as they update their "status" on social media by sharing current thoughts and feelings, they are going to complete a "status update" to open the session. This will give them an opportunity to briefly share what is going on in their life and what they are currently interested in. This status update can then be discussed and used to build rapport as well as open the session based on the information provided by the individual. Consider starting the discussion with some of the topics that tend to be of more interest to the individual such as "Listening to" and "Watching," and build rapport discussing these before beginning discussion on some of the other topics such as "Feeling" and "Thinking about."

Variations of the activity

- If completing the activity in a group session, allow each individual to share one of the items from his or her status update.
- If group time allows, the group could go through item by item and share and discuss each individual's responses.

Status Update Handout

Listening to. . . . .

. . . .

Watching. . . . .

. . . .

Looking up. . . . .

. . . .

Thinking about. . . . .

. . . .

Wishing for. . . . .

. . . .

Dreaming . . . .

. . . .

Feeling . . . .

. . . .

Up next for me. . . . .

. . . .

Posted by (name) . . . . on (date) . . . .

LIKE, DISLIKE, SHARE

Purpose of the activity

- To build rapport and put the individual at ease
- To identify positive and negative aspects of the individual's day as well as potential topics for discussion during the session
- To assist individual in becoming more aware of his thoughts and interests

Materials needed

- Copies of the Like, Dislike, Share Handout
- Markers/pens

Description of the activity

Ask the individual if he is familiar with the "Like" and "Share" buttons on social media websites. If not, explain that the buttons allow a person to "like" different photos, status updates, and other items as well as to click the "share" button and share things with their friends. Give the individual the Like, Dislike, Share Handout and ask him to complete it by listing some of the things that he is currently liking and disliking as well as something that he would like to share with others. Consider completing a handout along with the individual to put him at ease. After completing the handout, discuss the individual's responses and use them to begin discussion for the session.

Variations of the activity

- This activity can also be completed as a group icebreaker. Each individual would tell the group about the response that he listed in the "Share" section and discuss the information. Individuals can also share about their likes and dislikes, as appropriate. For example, if an individual's dislikes include the names of other people, then it would not be appropriate to share within a group setting.

Like, Dislike, Share Handout

Like: . . . .

. . . .

. . . .

. . . .

Dislike: . . . .

. . . .

. . . .

. . . .

Share: . . . .

. . . .

. . . .

. . . .

PICTURE PERFECT

Purpose of the activity

- To put the individual at ease and build rapport
- To promote creative thinking
- To provide an opportunity for self-expression

Materials needed

- Blank paper
- Markers/crayons/pencils
- A variety of single object pictures cut from magazines (examples include flowers, birds, cars, trees, animals, etc.)
- Scissors
- Glue

Description of the activity

Provide each individual with a sheet of paper and one of the magazine pictures of a *single* object as well as the other materials. Explain to the individual that he can glue the single object picture anywhere he would like on his paper. Next, he is to envision the scene around the picture and draw it using the markers, crayons, or other supplies. After completing the activity, allow the individual to share his drawing.

Variations of the activity

This activity can be easily adapted to a group setting. When completing in a group setting, it works well to give each individual a picture of the same type of object. For example, give each individual a picture of a different variety of flower or different types of animals. After completing the activity, allow each individual to share his drawing.

Discussion questions

- What inspired you about your magazine picture?
- Tell me about your drawing.
- What did you think about this activity?
- What was challenging about the activity? What was easy about the activity?
- What skills did you have to use to complete the activity?

VISUAL GROUP CONTRACT

Purpose of the activity

- To set ground rules for the group
- To promote group unity
- To explain the purpose of the group and obtain commitment to participate from members

Materials needed

- Large piece of paper taped to the wall
- Markers

Description of the activity

Welcome all the members to the group. Explain to them that the group is a place to learn and share. If the group has a more specific purpose (such as anger control, addictions, social skills, etc.), discuss this purpose with the participants. Tell them that everyone should feel safe and free to participate in the group. In order to do this, they will need to set some ground rules. Using the questions below, come up with a set of agreed group ground rules. List these rules on the large piece of paper. Make sure the rules are specific and stated positively (i.e. "Listen while others are talking" instead of "Don't talk when others are talking"). After the group members agree to the rules, have each of them sign the visual group contract indicating their agreement and commitment to the ground rules. Keep the visual contract displayed in the group space and refer to it frequently so that group members remember the expectations for the group. Remind them that while it is extremely important that they keep information discussed during the group confidential, the counselor cannot guarantee that it will be kept confidential by all members.

Variations of the activity

- This activity could also be done during the first session with an individual client to set the stage for a productive counseling relationship and to define clear expectations.
- As part of the group activity, the group members could also identify names, symbols, or mascots for their group to create even more unity.

Discussion questions

- How can the group be a safe place for all the members?

- How can members show respect and concern for each other?

- How will members handle it if there is a disagreement or conflict?

- What do the group members want to gain from the group?

- What do the members need from each other to make the group a productive place?

- What should happen if a member does not respect or follow the rules that are developed today?

- How will information that is shared during the group be handled? What are the limits of confidentiality?

INTRODUCING ME AND YOU

Purpose of the activity

- To encourage rapport and cohesiveness among group members
- To develop listening and communication skills
- To learn about group members' likes and dislikes

Materials needed

- Copies of the Introducing Me and You Handout
- Markers

Description of the activity

Divide the group members into groups of two students. Explain to the group that they are going to be interviewing each other and introducing each other to the group. Give each member a copy of the Introducing Me and You Handout. Allow the small group approximately ten minutes to complete their interviews with each other (one member interviews the other and then they switch places). After each small group finishes, bring the whole group back together. Go around the room and ask each pair to introduce each other and say one interesting thing that they learned about their partner from the interview.

Variations of the activity

- This activity could also be completed in an individual session with the counselor and individual interviewing each other.

Discussion questions

- What skills did you have to use when you were asking your partner questions?
- What skills did you have to use when you were being interviewed?
- What was the easiest part of this activity? What was the most challenging part?
- What did you like most about this activity?
- Did you prefer being the person asking the interview questions or answering the questions? Why?

Introducing Me and You Handout

Name: . . . . Birthday: . . . .

Age: . . . . Grade:. . . . .

Number of brothers and sisters: . . . .

Pets: . . . . Home town:. . . . .

Favorite food: . . . .

Favorite candy: . . . .

Favorite TV shows/movies: . . . .

Favorite sports: . . . .

Favorite school subject: . . . .

Least favorite school subject: . . . .

Favorite holiday: . . . .

Favorite hobbies/activities: . . . .

What I want to be when I grow up . . . .

Best thing that happened to me today: . . . .

HASHTAG HAPPENINGS

Purpose of the activity

- To provide an opportunity for participants to express their feelings and thoughts in a familiar way

- To open the session by getting a "quick" check on the participants

- To start the session in a non-threatening manner

Materials needed

- Markers, writing utensils

- Copies of the Hashtag Happenings Handout

Description of the activity

Provide participants with copies of the Hashtag Happenings Handout. Ask if anyone is familiar with using "hashtags" on social media. Explain to them that hashtags are used on various social media sites to mark key words and phrases. Ask students to give a few examples of hashtag phrases they have seen or used. Tell them that are going to create a hashtag to describe their day or how they are feeling. After the participants have completed their hashtags, ask them to share these and explain how they selected their hashtags.

Variations of the activity

- If using the activity as part of a group, see if there are any patterns or similar phrases among group members. Discuss the hashtags each member chose to describe their day/ feelings.

- Create a group hashtag that reflects a common theme for the group. Use the hashtag to promote unity within the group.

Hashtag Happenings Handout

Name: . . . .   Date: . . . .

\#

. . . .

. . . .

. . . .

. . . .

Brief description or drawing to explain my hashtag:

SELFIE

Purpose of the activity

- To provide an opportunity for participants to express their thoughts and feelings in a familiar way
- To build rapport at the beginning of the session
- To promote positive thinking skills

Materials needed

- Copies of the Selfie Handout
- Markers, crayons, pencils

Description of the activity

Ask the participant if he has ever posted a "selfie" on a social media website. Ask him what the purpose is of posting a "selfie." Explain that many people post "selfies" to let others know what is going on with them, what they are doing, or how they are feeling at a particular moment. Ask the participant to create his own "selfie" using the Selfie Handout and art supplies to give an idea of what is going on with him and how he is feeling at this particular moment. After the participant completes the activity, discuss his "selfie" with him as a means for opening the session.

Variations of the activity

- This activity also works well in group settings.
- It can also make a great bulletin board or display using the heading "Selfie Snapshots."

Selfie Handout

A picture of: . . . . posted on:. . . . .

GIVE ME FIVE

Purpose of the activity

- To develop rapport and open the session in a non-threatening manner

- To build relationship with the participant

- To encourage self-expression and communication skills

Materials needed

- Construction paper

- Scissors

- Pencils/markers

Description of the activity

Ask the participant to trace his hand, cut it out, and "give you five" things that happened to him that day (or during the time period that the participant was last seen) by writing them on each of the fingers of his hand. After this has been completed, discuss each of the things that the participant listed on his hand.

Variations of the activity

- High Five: List five positive things that happened that day (or within the time period since the participant was last seen).

- Low Five: List five negative things that happened that day (or within the time period since the participant was last seen).

BEGINNINGS BOWL

Purpose of the activity

- To open the session in a non-threatening manner
- To develop rapport with the individual
- To learn about possible areas of discussion for the session

Materials needed

- Bowl or basket to place items
- Assorted small items that can be used to create a scene or tell a story. Examples include small action heroes, Matchbox cars, small houses or buildings, small people, blocks, rocks, etc. Toys from dollar stores and/or toys from fast food chains children's meals are great sources of items for the basket

Description of the activity

Place the bowl of items on the table with the participant at the beginning. Ask the participant to look through the items in the bowl, choose items that he likes or is drawn to, and create a story or scene with them. Whichever is desired or age appropriate, the participant could write a brief story about the items he chose or draw a picture to explain his story or scene. When the individual has finished, ask him to tell you about the scene or story that he created using his items from the basket. Listen for any themes about possible issues (such as anger, family relationships, conflicts, social issues, etc.) that may be areas for discussion in the session.

Variations of the activity

- Partner Stories—this activity can work well in groups. Divide the group into pairs and ask each pair to create a scene or story using a selection of items from the basket. When complete, each pair can tell the group about their scene or story.

Discussion questions

- How did you select which items to include in your scene or story?
- Tell me about the scene you created with your items.
- How did you create your scene or story?
- What is happening in your scene or story?
- How are the people getting along in your scene or story?
- How will your scene or story end?

- What did you like about this activity?
- What was challenging about this activity?
- Did you notice any themes or ideas in your scene or story? If so, what were they?

If using Partner Stories:

- How did you and your partner work together to create the scene or story?
- What did you like about working with your partner on your scene or story?
- What was challenging about working with another person to create the scene or story?

CHAPTER 2

Shape It Up Series

THINKING OUTSIDE THE BOX AND BOXED IN

Purpose of the activity

- To introduce therapeutic topics in a non-threatening manner
- To promote self-expression
- To discuss patterns of getting "stuck" and ways to change patterns of thinking

Materials needed

- Copies of the Thinking Outside the Box and Boxed In Handout
- Markers, crayons, pens
- Scissors
- Glue
- Magazines, other materials for making a collage

Description of the activity

Ask the participant if she has ever heard the expressions "boxed in" or "thinking outside the box." If the participant has heard these expressions, ask her to tell you what they mean. "Boxed in" tends to be associated with being stuck in a box, feeling trapped, and a lack of forward progress. "Thinking outside the box" often means exploring new ways of doing things, changing old patterns, or looking at a different way of doing things. Ask the participant to think of a current issue or situation that she has been dealing with. In the square on the handout and using either markers, crayons, collage materials, or a combination, ask the participant to depict ways that she is "stuck" or struggling with the situation. Next, ask her to "think outside the box" and generate some new solutions and ways of thinking about the issue and then draw, make a collage, or use a combination of these to represent the possible solutions around the outside of the square on the handout. After the activity is complete, discuss the information from the participant's handout.

Variations of the activity

- This activity could be completed using small cardboard boxes. On the inside of the box, the individual could draw or collage the things that keep her "boxed in" and on the outside she could draw or collage ways to "think outside the box."

Discussion questions

- Tell me about what is inside your square and what influenced you to put it on the inside of your square.
- How long have you been dealing with the issue?
- What does it feel like to feel to be "boxed in"?
- What was it like to "think outside the box" about your issue?
- What are the pros and cons of some of the "outside the box" solutions you generated?
- What are some steps that you can take to implement some of your ideas and get out of the box?
- What might be some of the challenges as you move forward?
- What are some steps you will need to take to keep yourself from getting "boxed in" in the future?
- What did you learn today?

Thinking Outside the Box
and Boxed In Handout

OVAL OFFICE

Purpose of the activity

- To understand the importance of responsibility and organization
- To use creative thinking skills and express thoughts in a positive manner
- To discuss respect for authority figures

Materials needed

- Copies of the Oval Office Handout
- Markers, crayons, writing utensils

Description of the activity

Ask the participant if she knows what the Oval Office is (the office of the President of the United States). Discuss the many responsibilities of the President and all the things that he has to do in his office each day. Tell the participant that she is going to imagine that she is the President for the day and can arrange the Oval Office any way she wants. Give her a copy of the Oval Office Handout and ask her to create her own Oval Office. Tell her to consider all the things that she will need to do in her office and to be sure to create a space where she can work productively. After she completes the activity, use the discussion questions below to talk about responsibility, organization, and respect for authority.

Variations of the activity

- This is a great activity to be completed for President's Day. Cut out the students' Oval Offices and use them as a bulletin board display.

Discussion questions

- What would be the best thing about being President?
- What would be the most difficult thing about being President?
- Tell me about the Oval Office that you designed and why you chose each of the things in your office.
- What types of things does the President have to do in his office?
- What would happen if the President didn't have an office?
- What are some of the responsibilities of the President?
- What would happen if the President didn't take his responsibilities seriously?
- Why should people respect the President?
- Does respect have to be earned?

- What are some of the things that you have to keep organized?

- What happens when you don't keep things organized in your bookbag, desk, etc?

- What are some of your responsibilities?

- What happens when you don't take your responsibilities seriously?

- How can we look at the things you put in your Oval Office and come up with a plan for better organization and responsibility for your current roles?

Oval Office Handout

Design your own Oval Office

WE'RE ALL STARS

Purpose of the activity

- To promote positive thinking
- To encourage group unity
- To develop social skills

Materials needed

- Copies of the We're All Stars Handout
- Pencils, pens
- Markers, crayons
- Scissors

Description of the activity

Ask the group if they have ever heard the expression "all star" used. Explain that it is frequently used in sports to describe the best players or a team made up of the very best players. Actors and actresses are often called stars, too, because other people are very interested in them. Tell the group that each group member is also an "all star." Ask each participant to write his or her name decoratively in the center of the star. Tell them that they are going to pass their star to the person sitting to their right. The person sitting to their right will write something positive about the individual whose name is on the star in one of the five points of the star. Continue passing the stars until all of the participants have something written in each of the points of their star. When the stars get back around to the person whose name is in the center, ask the individual to write a positive statement about him or herself underneath the star. Discuss the activity with the group using the discussion questions below. Explain to them that they are "all stars." If time allows, let participants color and cut out their stars.

Variations of the activity

- For an individual activity, the counselor can write positive statements on the star and discuss these with the participant. Positive statements could also be obtained from others, such as parents and teachers.
- This makes a great bulletin board when the stars are cut out and laminated with the title "We're All Stars."

Discussion questions

- Was it easier to write nice things about yourself or others?
- What was the best thing about this activity?

- What was the most challenging thing about this activity?
- How did it feel to read the nice things that others wrote about you?
- What does it mean to be an "all star?"
- Did anyone write something on your paper that surprised you or that you didn't know about yourself?
- What does it feel like to receive a compliment from others?
- What does it feel like to give a compliment to others?
- Why is it important to say kind things to others?

We're All Stars Handout

ME MADE OUT OF SHAPES

Purpose of the activity

- To encourage creativity and self-expression
- To develop positive self-image and positive thinking skills
- To promote communication skills and social skills

Materials needed

- Scissors
- Glue
- Construction paper cut-outs of various shapes in different sizes (examples: small circles, triangles, squares for facial features; large rectangles, triangles, squares, circles for body parts)

Description of the activity

Tell the participant that she is going to create a self-portrait of herself using the various shapes available. Explain to her that she can combine the shapes in any way that she wants to make the portrait. While the individual is completing the activity, discuss the importance of self-talk and thinking positive thoughts about herself. After the self-portrait is complete, encourage the participant to talk about the portrait and say why she chose the combination of shapes that she did. Next, assist the participant in identifying some of the thoughts she may struggle with (examples might be "Nobody likes me," "I am not very smart," "I act up") and in developing positive statements to think instead (such as "I am a friendly person," "I am smart and capable," "I can control my actions"). Ask the participant to write some of these phrases on the shapes that make up the self-portrait. Ask her to display the self-portrait in a prominent place and work on using the positive statements instead of the negative ones.

Variations of the activity

- This activity also works well in a group setting.

Discussion questions

- Tell me about your self-portrait.
- What are some "negative" thoughts or things you may think about yourself?
- What are some positive thoughts and phrases that you could use to replace the "negative" thoughts?
- How does it impact you when your thinking is negative?
- How does it impact you when your thinking is positive?
- What are some strategies that you can use to focus on positive thoughts?
- Where can you display your self-portrait so that you are reminded about the positive statements we identified today?

ON MY HEART NOW

Purpose of the activity

- To promote creativity and self-expression
- To learn to express thoughts and feelings in a positive manner
- To develop communication skills

Materials needed

- Copies of the On My Heart Now Handout
- Scissors
- Glue
- Old magazines with a variety of pictures/collage materials

Description of the activity

Ask participants to think about some expressions that people may say using the word "heart." Examples may include "I love you with all my heart," "That breaks my heart," and "I have you on my heart right now." Talk with the students about these expressions and what they mean. Many people consider the "heart" to be the center of our being from which life flows. Ask the participants to think about some things that they "love with all their hearts" and "some things that are on their hearts." Distribute the materials and ask the participants to find pictures and symbols to represent these things and then glue them on the heart on the handout. Participants can cut out their hearts when they are finished. When all the participants are finished, allow them to share their hearts and talk about the images and symbols they selected.

Variations of the activity

- This works well as an individual activity that can be completed one on one with the participant and counselor.
- This is a great activity for Valentine's Day. A display could be created using the hearts with a title such as "Our Hearts are Full of Love."

On My Heart Now Handout

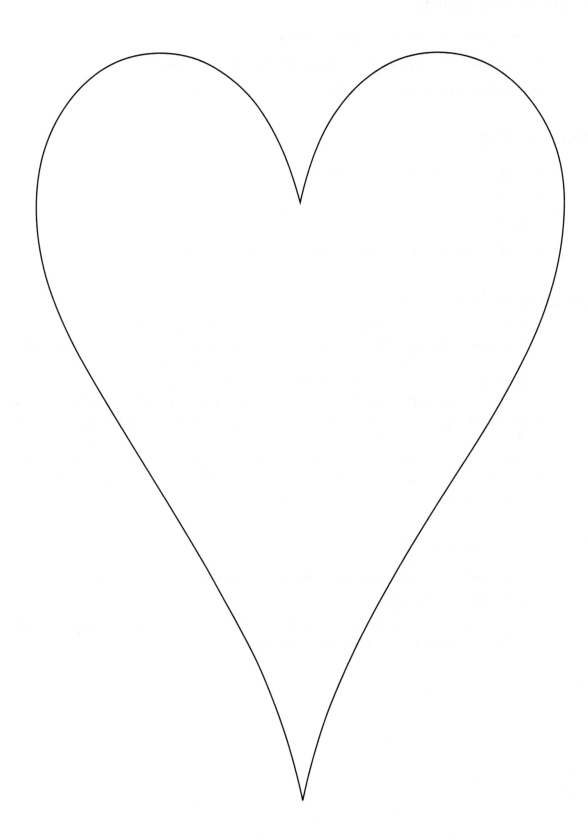

GOING IN CIRCLES

Purpose of the activity

- To discuss ways that individuals "get stuck" in patterns of behavior and thought
- To identify ways to change behaviors
- To promote self-expression and creativity

Materials needed

- Paper
- Washable paint
- Paint brushes
- Bowl for paint
- Markers
- Empty paper towel holders or other small circular-shaped objects

Description of the activity

Discuss with the participant the expression "I am just going in circles." What do people mean by this expression? Most people mean that they are in a pattern of doing the same thing over and over again. Ask the participant to identify some things that she seems to be "going in circles" about in her life. Assist her in identifying some possible changes that could be made to stop "going in circles" in that area of her life. Explain to her that she is going to create a piece of art to assist her in remembering the concepts discussed. Give the participant a piece of paper and pour some black paint in the bowl. Ask her to dip the end of the paper towel holder in the paint and then press it down repeatedly over the paper to make a pattern of circles. This can be done as she chooses, with circles overlapping or not overlapping. Allow the paint to dry and then the participant can fill in the white space between the circles with either paint or markers in a variety of colors to create a beautiful piece of art. As the participant works, continue to discuss various ways to change and improve behavior.

Variations of the activity

- This also works well as a group activity.
- A compass tool could be used to create a variety of circles on the paper.

MANDALAS OF MINDFULNESS

Purpose of the activity

- To promote positive thinking and healthy emotional regulation
- To encourage self-esteem and self-awareness
- To develop coping skills

Materials needed

- Blank CDs (no writing on at least one side of the CD)
- Sharpie (fine point) markers (these can be used on more surfaces such as plastic, wood, etc.)
- Paper
- Puff paint
- Paint markers or acrylic paint
- Rulers
- Images/examples of mandalas (www.mandalaproject.org has some great examples)
- Small circular coins, buttons, or similar materials for the participant to trace (if needed)

Description of the activity

Begin by showing the participants images of the mandalas. Ask if any of the participants have ever seen images like these or know what they are called. Explain that the images are pictures of mandalas. Mandala is the Sanskrit word for circle, but it also emphasizes wholeness and balance in life. Many people use mandalas as part of meditation and as a means of focusing their attention on something positive. Mandalas can also encourage mindfulness. Mindfulness means to be aware of one's thoughts, feelings, and emotions as well as to stay focused on the present moment. Mandalas can provide the participants with a means to remember to be mindful and provide something positive to focus their attention on in the present moment.

Mandalas have a center point from which the pattern radiates out (typically in a symmetrical manner). Distribute the needed materials to each participant. Using the ruler, ask each participant to draw black lines with the Sharpie marker to divide his or her mandala into either four or eight equal size sections. Ask the participants to create a symmetrical and repeating pattern in each of the sections using the ruler, small circular coins, and other desired shapes with the Sharpie marker. Once the pattern is complete, participants can use the black puff paint to trace over their black Sharpie lines. This will need to dry (preferably overnight) before proceeding on to the next step. The puff paint creates a raised line or border for the design. Once the puff paint has dried, ask the participants to select four or five colors to fill in the design on the mandala. After the participants have completed the mandalas, share them with the group and discuss ways that they may use their mandalas.

Variations of the activity

- In settings where more brief activities are needed, the entire project could be completed using colored Sharpie markers instead of paint.

- In group settings with more extended time periods, the group can create a collaborative mandala on a large circle. This can become a wonderful display in the group space.

- Mandalas can be arranged into beautiful displays by connecting them with yarn and hanging them from the ceiling or a window.

Discussion questions

- What does it mean to be "whole" or "complete?"

- How is the mandala a symbol of wholeness and balance?

- What does it mean to have balance in your life?

- How do you feel when things are out of balance in your life?

- How do you get things back in balance?

- How could the mandala help you focus your attention?

- What does it mean to be mindful?

- How can you stay aware of your feelings and emotions?

- What does it mean to stay focused on the present moment?

- What are some ways that you can encourage mindfulness in your life?

- Why do you think people have used mandalas as part of meditation and focusing attention on something positive throughout the centuries?

- How will you use the mandala you created in your personal life?

- What was the experience of creating the mandala like for you?

DIAMOND IN THE ROUGH

Purpose of the activity

- To promote positive thinking skills
- To encourage self-esteem and identify positive traits in self
- To develop communication skills and goal-setting skills

Materials needed

- Copies of the Diamond in the Rough Handout
- Magazines, collage materials
- Markers, pencils
- Glue
- Scissors

Description of the activity

Ask the participant if she has ever heard the expression "a diamond in the rough." Explain that this expression is used to describe someone with wonderful qualities and potential that are hidden or not easily observed by others at the present time. Diamonds are beautiful stones but they may be hidden among rock. Discuss some individuals who may have been "diamonds in the rough" in the past, but continued to work to reach their full potential. Examples include:

- Michael Jordan—was deemed too short for the varsity basketball team, before becoming a famous professional basketball player.
- Walt Disney—fired from his job at a newspaper for lacking ideas, but went on to become a famous and innovative filmmaker and amusement park developer.
- J.K. Rowling—at times jobless, and whose bestselling *Harry Potter* series was rejected by 12 publishing houses before eventually being accepted.
- Jay-Z—could not get a record deal and was selling CDs out of his car before becoming a famous rapper and starting his own label.
- Bill Gates—dropped out of college and failed at his first business attempt before co-founding Microsoft.
- Oprah Winfrey—endured abuse and was demoted from her job as a news anchor before starting her talk show and television network.
- The Beatles—rejected by multiple record labels before going on to become one of the most famous bands of all times.

Provide the participant with a copy of the Diamond in the Rough Handout and other necessary supplies. Ask her to think about some of the "hidden potential" in her and some of the "diamond in the rough" experiences in her life. Ask her to make a collage about this on the handout. Discuss it when complete.

Variations of the activity

- If time allows, the diamond shape could be made using cardboard and then covered in tin foil to create a shiny background before gluing on the collage images.

- This is also great as a group activity. A display can be created with the heading "We are Sparkling Diamonds."

Discussion questions

- What does it mean to be a "diamond in the rough?"

- How do you feel when others do not see your positive qualities and potential?

- What are some ways to stay positive and keep trying, even when others reject you or do not give you a chance?

- Were you surprised at any of the famous individuals who were "diamonds in the rough?"

- What is a personal trait or quality that might be "hidden potential" within you?

- How do you work to develop your hidden potential?

- What are a few reasons not to give up when others do not see your potential right away?

- What would have happened to the famous people if they had not kept trying?

- What will be a goal for you in developing your "hidden potential" and focusing on your positive traits?

Diamond in the Rough Handout

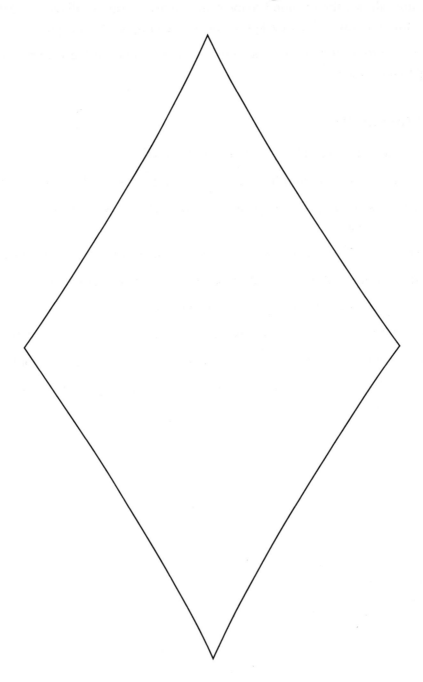

A goal to develop my hidden potential: . . . .

. . . .

A positive statement about my potential: . . . .

. . . .

COMPLETING THE CIRCLE

Purpose of the activity

- To build group unity and cohesiveness
- To promote self-expression and communication skills
- To increase social skills

Materials needed

- Copies of the Completing the Circle Handout
- Markers or crayons
- Scissors
- Glue
- Construction paper

Description of the activity

Discuss social skills and unity with the group. Discuss the benefits of talking with others about issues and sharing thoughts with a supportive group. Discuss the unique qualities that each person brings to the group. Explain that the group will be working together to create a circle(s) that represents the group. Divide the group into smaller groups of four. If there are not even numbers, the group leader can complete one as well, or group members may volunteer to do more than one quarter of the circle. Cut the circle on the Completing the Circle Handout into four equal sections. Give each participant one of the four sections. Ask each small group to work together to select four or five colors (this gives a look of cohesiveness) to use on their parts of the circle. Each participant can design his or her portion of the circle as he or she wishes using the colors that the group selects. After each individual has completed a section, the group can work together to arrange the four parts into a whole circle and then glue the circle to the piece of construction paper.

Variations of the activity

- This activity works well as an icebreaker or opening activity for new groups.
- This makes a fun display or bulletin board using the heading "We're All Part of the Circle."

Discussion questions

- What are the advantages of being part of a group?
- What does it mean to have group unity?
- Why is group unity important?
- What are some of the positive qualities that each member brings to the group?

- What would the circle be like if one of the parts was missing?

- What was your experience of working in the group to create the circle?

- How did your small group select colors and put the individual parts together into the whole circle?

- How do you feel about being part of the group?

Completing the Circle Handout

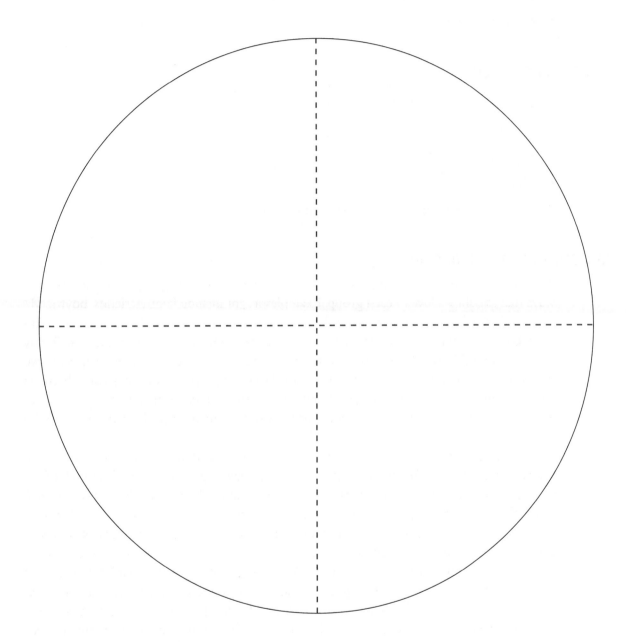

LOVE TRIANGLE

Purpose of the activity

- To identify healthy ways to show love to self and others

- To increase self-awareness and self-esteem

- To promote coping skills

Materials needed

- Copies of the Love Triangle Handout

- Markers, crayons

- Scissors

- Glue

- Collage materials (images from magazines, etc.)

Description of the activity

Ask the participant how she defines love. Discuss different people/groups that she loves and ways that she shows love to each group. Examples might include family, friends, boyfriend/girlfriend, self. Ask if the participant has ever heard the expression "love triangle." This expression is often used to describe an out-of-balance relationship. For example, a male may be in a relationship with two females at the same time, or a female in a relationship with two males at the same time. This makes the relationship complicated and creates issues between all three individuals in the triangle. Similarly, it can be complicated to keep a balance between the individuals in different areas of life and to maintain healthy relationships with different groups.

Give the individual three copies of the Love Triangle Handout. On the first triangle, ask the participant to write the three most important groups of people in her life at each of the three points on the triangle. For example, an individual might list friends, family, and self, or boyfriend, best friend, and mom. Ask the individual to choose one color for each person or group. Ask her to color a portion of the triangle to represent the amount of time and energy that she currently invests in the relationship with each person. For example, if she listed friends, family, and self, she might color a large portion of the triangle in the color chosen for friends if she spends a great deal of time and energy on her relationships with her friends and then smaller segments for self and family if she spends less time on these two areas. On the second triangle, ask her to use the same three colors to represent each group or individual, but this time to draw out the ideal balance (if this is different from the current balance in her life). For example, if the individual wishes she had more time to spend with her dad and to take care of herself, then she might reduce the amount for friends and increase the sections for family and self. On the third triangle, allow the participant to make a collage, or draw or write healthy ways to show love to each group or individual that she listed at each point of the triangle. Discuss each of the triangles with her.

Variations of the activity

- This can be a helpful activity for children of divorced or separated parents.

Discussion questions

- What is your definition of love?

- How do you show love to others?

- Is the type of love you have for family different from the love you have for friends? How?

- Do you show love to different groups and individuals in different ways?

- How do you determine how you spend your time and energy in the different relationships in your life?

- How do you feel about the current relationships in your life and how your time is spent in each relationship?

- What does it feel like when your relationships are out of balance or you are not getting along with people who you care about?

- Have you ever felt caught between two people who you have relationships with? How did you handle it?

- What are your concerns about your relationships at this time?

- What is going well with your relationships at this time?

- What changes would you like to make in your current relationships?

- How can you achieve more balance in your relationships?

- What are some new and different ways to show others that you care about them?

- What are some ways that you can show love to yourself and take care of yourself in your relationships with others?

- How did completing this activity make you feel?

Love Triangle Handout

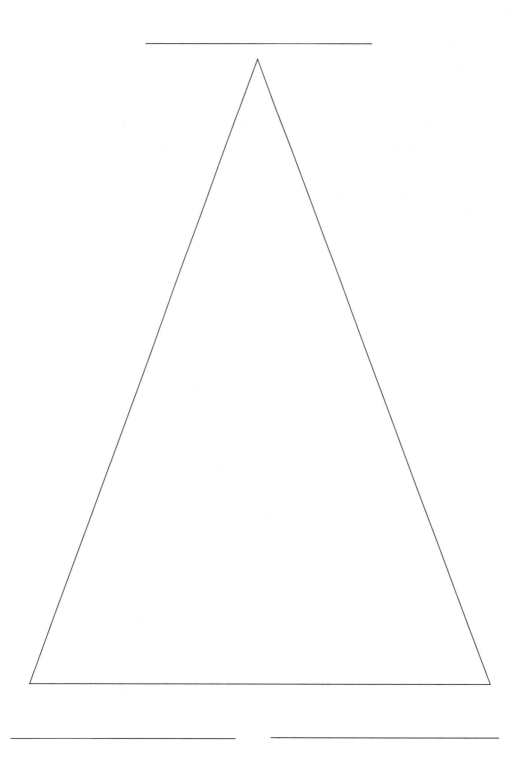

REACHING FOR OUR STARS

Purpose of the activity

- To promote positive thinking and coping skills
- To encourage goal setting
- To develop communication skills and promote self-expression

Materials needed

- Copies of the Reaching for Our Stars Handout (copy on yellow paper if possible)
- Construction paper
- Scissors
- Glue
- Markers, pencils
- Large piece of paper with "Reaching for Our Stars" written across the top

Description of the activity

Ask the participants if they have ever heard the expression "reach for the stars." This usually means to set goals high or to work toward big goals. Discuss with the group that goals tend to be different from person to person. One person may have a goal to become a teacher, one may want to become a doctor, one may want to be a basketball player, and so on. Just as each person is a unique individual, each person's goals will be unique as well. Give each participant a copy of the Reaching for Our Stars Handout. Ask them to think of a long-term goal in their life. Ask the participants to write the goal in the center of their stars and then decorate the star as desired. Once complete, ask the individuals to cut out the stars and attach them to the top of the large piece of paper under the words "Reaching for Our Stars." After all the participants have done this, ask them to think of some steps that they will need to take to reach their goals. For example, if someone wants to be a teacher, he or she would need to graduate high school, go to college, and gain experience working with children/teens, etc. If someone wanted to be a basketball player, he or she would need to play for high school leagues, practice frequently, and go to camps and clinics, etc. Distribute a piece of construction paper to each participant. Ask participants to trace their hand and the bottom part of their arm on the construction paper and then cut it out. Ask them to write their name on the arm part and then list five steps that they would need to take to reach "their" star and then decorate it as desired. When complete, ask each participant to attach his or her star to the large piece of paper. This makes a beautiful display.

Variations of the activity

- This can also be done as an individual activity by changing the name to "Reaching for My Star" and using a smaller piece of paper.

Discussion questions

- What does it mean to reach for the stars?
- What is a goal that you have set for yourself?
- What are you doing now so that you can reach your goal?
- What future steps will you need to take to reach your goal?
- What positive thoughts can you use to stay motivated about working toward your goal?
- How can you encourage others to work toward their goals?
- How will you handle it if you have a setback in your progress toward your goal?
- Who will be your support system in reaching your goal?
- What will you do to celebrate progress toward your goal?

Reaching for Our Stars Handout

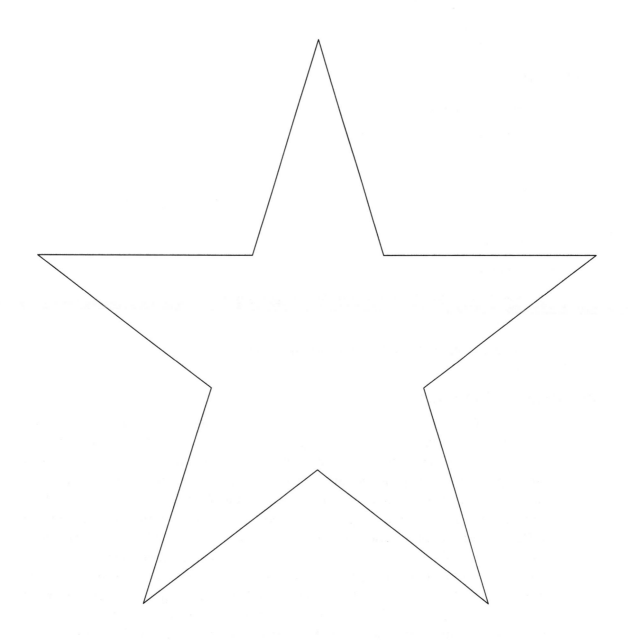

STAR DUST

Purpose of the activity

- To promote positive thinking
- To build coping skills
- To encourage self-esteem

Materials needed

- Colored sidewalk chalk
- Ziploc bags
- Hammer or mallet
- Glitter
- Water
- Small bowls
- Paint brushes
- Construction paper or cardstock (heavy-weight) paper
- Markers
- Optional: completed Reaching for Our Stars banner

Description of the activity

Before the individuals arrive, place sidewalk chalk in the Ziploc bags and crush into a fine powder using the hammer, mallet, or rolling pin. Place each of the different colors of chalk into a small bowl. When the individuals arrive, explain that the activity today will be a follow-up to the Reaching for Our Stars activity. Explain to the group that when working toward a long-term goal or dealing with something difficult, visual reminders and symbols of encouragement are needed along the way. Since the individuals completed the Reaching for Our Stars activity at the last session, explain that today they will be making "Star dust" to serve as a visual reminder to them to keep sparkling and reaching toward their goals. Distribute paper to each participant. Allow the participants to select the color of the crushed sidewalk chalk that they would like to use. Assist them in adding the desired amount of glitter to the crushed sidewalk chalk. Next, help them to slowly add water to the paint and glitter mixture until it reaches a paint-like consistency. Be careful not to add too much water or the mixture will become too thin. Provide the individuals with a paint brush (or they can use their fingers to finger paint) and ask them to use the "star dust" to create star dust art on their paper. Allow the "star dust" art to dry and then have the individuals write "Star Dust" on the top of the paper as well as a positive affirmation that is meaningful to them. These can serve as a visual reminder to remain positive when facing obstacles and to continue working toward their goals.

Variation of the activity

- If the group created the Reaching for Our Stars banner, then each participant could paint the "star dust" flowing down from their star at the top of the banner to their arm print. When dry, the individuals can write a positive affirmation along their "star dust."

- If time does not allow for the painting activity, the "star dust" could be created by crushing the sidewalk chalk, placing it in a Ziploc bag, and adding the glitter. The individuals could create a label to enclose in the bag that states "star dust" and lists a positive affirmation that is meaningful to the them.

Discussion questions

- What did we do in the last session as part of the Reaching for Our Stars activity?

- What did you learn from that activity?

- Why is it important to think positively about our goals and ourselves?

- How can you promote positive thinking in your life?

- What is a positive affirmation?

- How can you use positive affirmations when faced with a challenge or difficulty?

- Why is it important to have visual reminders of positive statements and images, and reminders of our goals around us?

- What can you do when you have a negative thought or start to doubt yourself?

- Where can you display your "star dust" art to remind you to think positively and stay on the path to your goal?

BACK TO SQUARE 1

Purpose of the activity

- To develop self-esteem and positive self-concept
- To encourage creativity and self-expression
- To develop skills in following directions

Materials needed

- Copies of the Back to Square 1 Handout
- Markers, crayons, colored pencils

Description of the activity

Ask the participants if they have ever heard the expression "back to square 1." Explain that this expression means to go back to the beginning or back to basics. Explain to the students that they are going to complete a "back to basics" activity that will give some basic information about themselves in a creative way as well as help them to practice their listening skills and skills in following direction. Provide each participant with a copy of the Back to Square 1 Handout and writing/drawing supplies.

Ask the participants to draw or write the following in the appropriately numbered square. Pause in between calling out each item to give participants time to complete the task. When finished, discuss the activity with the participants.

Information to be written or drawn in each square:

1. first name or initial (written as decoratively as the participant chooses)
2. favorite color (color the entire square with favorite color)
3. birth date
4. favorite shape
5. drawing of favorite hobby
6. age
7. drawing of favorite food
8. middle name or initial (written as decoratively as the participant chooses)
9. number of siblings
10. drawing of favorite animal
11. last name or initial (written as decoratively as the participant chooses)
12. drawing of favorite season

13. color (color the square any color you choose)

14. favorite number

15. drawing of favorite sport

16. drawing of favorite holiday.

Discussion questions

- What was the easiest part of this activity?

- What was the most difficult part of this activity?

- How did this activity help you practice listening and following directions?

- What would happen if you did not listen during the activity?

- What are some ways to improve your listening skills in other settings?

- What are some ways to improve your ability to follow directions in other settings?

Variations of the activity

- If completed in a group, a prize could be given for the participant who best followed directions.

- These could be used as bingo cards for an All about Me bingo game.

Back to Square 1 Handout

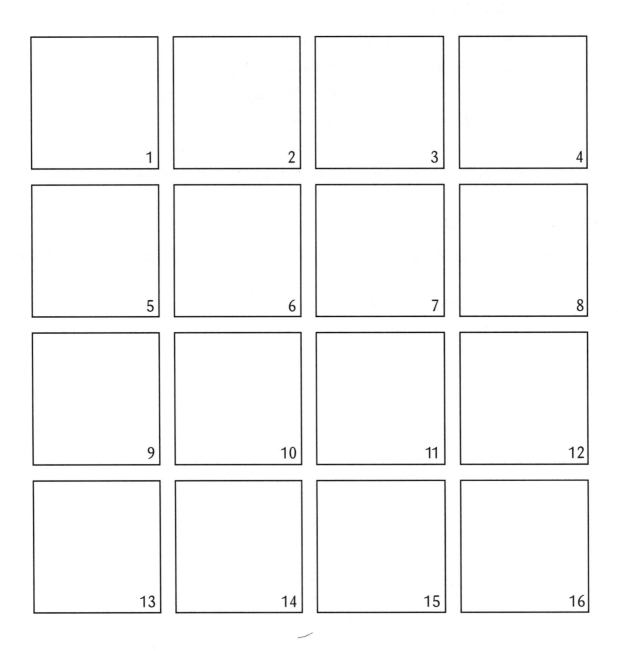

1	2	3	4
5	6	7	8
9	10	11	12
13	14	15	16

WHAT GETS ME BENT OUT OF SHAPE?

Purpose of the activity

- To identify triggers for anger and frustration

- To identify positive coping skills

- To encourage communication skills

Materials needed

- Copies of the What Gets Me Bent out of Shape? Handout

- Markers, crayons, pencils

- Index cards or other small sized paper (if completing the variation)

Description of the activity

Ask the participant if she has ever heard the expression "getting bent out of shape." Explain to her that this expression means to get angry, frustrated, or upset. Ask the participant to think of some things that get her "bent out of shape." This could be certain activities, situations, individuals, or anything else that triggers her to become upset. Provide the individual with a copy of the What Gets Me Bent out of Shape? Handout. Ask her to draw or write about the things that get her "bent out of shape." When complete, discuss these triggers for frustration and anger and help her to identify ways to cope with each of the triggers.

Variations of the activity

- This activity also works well with groups. It can be interesting to see what common triggers there are among group members.

- Group members can make a "What To Do When I'm Getting Bent Out of Shape" index card that they can keep in their pockets or at their desks to remind them of coping and anger management strategies when they feel angry or upset. Examples of strategies that individuals might list on their card include asking for a break to cool down, moving away from others, and taking deep breaths.

Discussion questions

- What were some of the triggers that you identified that make you feel frustrated, angry, or upset?

- What are some coping and anger management strategies that you can use when you start to feel angry or upset?

- Is there a way to reduce your exposure to certain things that may trigger anger or frustration? If so, how?

- What are some of the signs that you are beginning to become frustrated or angry? Examples might include clenched fists, feeling hot, and gritting teeth.

- What steps can you take when you start to notice or feel these signs in your body to prevent your anger from escalating?

- Why is it important to know the triggers for your anger and frustration?

- How can it help you to use your coping skills instead of becoming angry?

What Gets Me Bent out of Shape? Handout

Make a list or draw examples of activities, events, or other things that may trigger you to become angry, frustrated, or upset.

GETTING IN SHAPE

Purpose of the activity

- To promote positive self-concept
- To develop coping skills
- To identify ways to be healthy in all aspects of self

Materials needed

- Copies of the Getting in Shape Handout
- Collage materials (magazines and other sources of images)
- Glue
- Scissors
- Pencils, markers, pens

Description of the activity

Ask the individual if she has ever heard anyone use the expression "I am going to get in shape." Explain that many people use this expression to mean that they are going to get physically healthy by exercising and eating well. While it is important to take care of our physical health, it is also important to be mentally and emotionally healthy. Provide the participant with a copy of the Getting in Shape Handout as well as collage materials. Ask her to select images that show how to become physically healthy, emotionally healthy, and mentally healthy and then glue them to the appropriate section of the handout. The participant may also choose to draw or write about each section. After the activity is complete, discuss the images and responses that the participant gave and, if needed, help her to identify additional ways to stay healthy in each area.

Variations of the activity

- This activity is a good one to use in January when many people focus on New Year's resolutions and "getting in shape."

Discussion questions

- What does it mean to "get in shape?"
- What are some ways to take care of yourself and stay healthy physically?
- What are some ways to take care of yourself and stay healthy mentally?
- What are some ways to take care of yourself and stay healthy emotionally?
- Why is it important to engage in "self-care" and stay healthy?

- What are some signs or symptoms that may indicate that you need to engage in some "self-care" strategies? Examples might include feeling tired all the time, overeating or loss of appetite, not feeling well, isolating yourself, etc.

- Why is it important to not neglect any of the aspects of your health—physical, emotional or mental?

- What is one new strategy or approach that you can implement in each area of health (physical, emotional, mental) in your life?

Getting in Shape Handout

Physical health:

Emotional health:

Mental health:

CHAPTER 3

Visual and Expressive Arts Activities

A DAY IN MY SHOES
Purpose of the activity

- To develop positive self-concept
- To encourage communication skills
- To express thoughts and feelings in a creative manner

Materials needed

- Paper
- Pencils, markers, crayons
- Collage images (old magazines, etc.)
- Scissors
- Glue

Description of the activity

Ask the participant if he has ever heard anyone use the expression "walk a mile in my shoes." The expression means that before we judge others or criticize others, we must try to consider the difficulties and challenges that they have faced. One word for this is empathy. Others should also consider the difficulties and challenges that the participant has faced before judging the individual. Distribute the supplies to the individual. Ask the participant to trace one or both of his shoes, depending on the size of his feet and the size of the paper. Inside the traced shape, ask the participant to make a collage or draw a picture about what it is like to walk a day in his shoes, about some of the difficulties and challenges he has faced, and how others can better understand him. When complete, ask the participant to tell you about the images and drawings he included and what they mean.

Variations of the activity

- This is also a great group activity. It can help group members understand the concept of empathy and relate to one another, and it can build group unity.

- This makes a great display. The participants can cut out their shoeprints and then a banner can be created with the title "Walk a Mile in Our Shoes."

Discussion questions

- What does the expression "walk a mile my shoes" mean?

- Why should we not judge or criticize others?

- What does it mean to have empathy for others?

- Can you ever really understand the experiences that someone else has had? Why or why not?

- How can you show empathy for others?

- How can you help others understand the experiences that you've had?

- How do you handle it if someone does judge or criticize you?

- What are some positive ways to cope with judgment and criticism from others?

- Tell me about the images and drawings you included in your shoeprint.

- How have your experiences, challenges, and difficulties shaped you?

- How did you feel about this activity?

- What did you learn about yourself as part of this activity?

- What did you learn about others in the group? Were there any shared or similar experiences between group members?

- What are some of the ways that you have coped with difficulties and challenges in your life?

- What do you want others to know and understand about you?

A LETTER ABOUT ME

Purpose of the activity

- To promote positive self-concept
- To express thoughts and feelings in a creative and positive manner
- To build rapport and a relationship with the counselor

Materials needed

- Paper
- Pencils
- Scissors
- Markers
- Colored pencils

Description of the activity

Tell the participant that today he is going to create a "letter" about himself. Ask him to trace the first letter of his name in a block style format. For younger participants, you may choose to do this ahead of time. The letter should be done in a block style with open space inside so that there is space for the participant to draw. Explain to the participant that he can draw pictures and symbols, write words that describe himself, and design the inside of his letter as he chooses. Some individuals may be able to complete the activity without any further guidance, while some may need additional suggestions. Examples of things that participants might choose to include are images of their favorite sports, hobbies, pets, food, adjectives that describe them, or their birthday. When complete, the participant can cut out his letter. Once this is complete, ask the participant to tell you about his "Letter About Me" and the things that he chose to include.

Variations of the activity

- If time allows, the participant can create "A Letter about Me" for his last name also. The participant could include additional drawings, words, and symbols to describe himself on the letter for his last name. This is a good activity for a group to complete. The group members can each share their letters with the group to build group unity and help group members relate to each other.

- These make a great display. They can be displayed using the heading "All About Me in Letters" or a hole can be punched in the top of the letter and they can be hung with yarn or string around the room.

Discussion questions

- What did you draw or write in your letter to explain about yourself?
- What does your letter tell us about you?
- What would you like others to know about you?
- What did you like about this activity?
- What is your favorite thing about yourself?
- What is something new that you learned about one of the other group members?
- What is something that you have in common with someone in the group?
- Why is it important to take time to share about our likes, dislikes, and things about ourselves?
- Why is it important to learn about other people?
- How can we learn from each other?

WE'RE ALL PIECES OF THE PUZZLE

Purpose of the activity

- To build group unity
- To develop rapport and a relationship among group members
- To promote self-expression and creativity

Materials needed

- Puzzle (with enough pieces for each group member to have one piece)
- White spray paint
- Acrylic or tempura paint
- Paint brushes
- Paper or board to attach puzzle
- Heavy duty glue to hold puzzle pieces

Description of the activity

In advance, spray paint the puzzle white and allow time for it to dry. Begin the discussion by telling the group members that everyone has an important part in the group and that each person brings unique and special qualities to the group as a whole. Explain that the group is much like a puzzle which is one big whole picture made up of many individual pieces. Distribute a puzzle piece to each group member to paint with colors and/or symbols that they like and that reflect their personality. After the pieces have been painted and dried, ask the group to work together to assemble the puzzle. Once assembled, the group can glue the puzzle to a board or a piece of paper. This can be framed or displayed in the group area as a reminder of the importance of the group and each member.

Variations of the activity

- This activity can also be done by creating your own puzzle. Using a large piece of paper or poster-board, create a puzzle by cutting puzzle pieces out of the paper. Distribute markers or paint to each group member to design their individual pieces. When complete the group members assemble the puzzle on a large bulletin board or wall space. This makes a great display with the heading "We're All Pieces of the Puzzle."

Discussion questions

- What is the purpose of a group?
- What are some of the unique things that you contribute to the group?
- What do you appreciate that others bring to the group?

- How is a puzzle like a group?

- Did everyone's puzzle piece look exactly the same? Why not?

- What would the puzzle look like if all the pieces were exactly the same?

- How should we treat other members in the group?

- How would you like other group members to treat you?

- What did you learn from this activity?

- What does a puzzle look like when it is put together? What does it look like when all the pieces are not assembled?

- Is the puzzle more meaningful when it is put together or taken apart?

TREE OF LIFE TIMELINE

Purpose of the activity

- To promote positive self-concept
- To build relationships and learn about an individual's perception of life events
- To develop coping skills and positive thinking skills

Materials needed

- Markers, crayons, pencils
- Pieces of poster-board or large paper
- Image of a cut tree trunk (www.arborday.org/trees/ringsLivingForest.cfm has a good picture and explanation of how the age of a tree is calculated)

Description of the activity

This is a fun variation on a timeline activity. Ask the group if anyone knows how the age of a tree can be calculated using the tree trunk. Explain that a tree's age is determined by counting the number of rings in the tree's trunk. We can also find out information about the tree's life by looking at the shape and color of the rings. Show the group some images of a tree trunk and its rings for visual inspiration. Distribute the supplies to each group member and explain that each person will be completing their own tree trunk timeline by drawing the number of rings to represent their age and then within each ring writing key words or drawing symbols to describe the events that happened in their life at that age. Rings could be done in different colors if desired by the group member. When the Tree of Life Timeline activity is complete, ask group members to share details about their timeline and tell the group some of the highlights that they included.

Variations of the activity

- This activity can be a great addition to a science lesson on trees or as an Arbor Day activity.
- This also works well as an activity to complete in an individual session.

Discussion questions

- What does a timeline tell us about a person?
- How can timelines and learning about a person's history help us to understand others?
- Tell me about your Tree of Life Timeline.

- How did you choose which events and parts of your life to include on your timeline?

- Does the shape or size of the rings on your timeline have any special meaning?

- What did you like about creating your timeline?

- What was challenging about creating your timeline?

- Do you think it is important to think about and understand some of the things that happened in your past? Why or why not?

- What did you learn about the other group members from their Tree of Life Timelines?

- What did you learn about yourself from this activity?

POSITIVE WORD ART

Purpose of the activity

- To develop positive thinking skills
- To promote healthy coping skills
- To encourage positive self-concept

Materials needed

- Art canvas or heavy-weight board/paper
- Painter's tape
- Paint
- Paint brushes

Description of the activity

Begin by discussing the importance of positive thinking with the individual and the need to surround oneself with positive thoughts, words, and images. Explain to the individual that today he is going to create some Positive Word Art. Allow the individual some time to think about a word or short phrase that reminds him to think positively. Examples might include hope, peace, love, trust, faith. Once the individual has chosen his word or phrase, spell out the word on the canvas using the painter's tape. Next, provide the participant with all the supplies and ask him to paint the entire canvas as he chooses, using colors that are positive to him. After the paint has dried, remove the painter's tape from the canvas. The positive word chosen by the individual will be white (the color of the canvas) with the paint all around it. The individual can take this project home with him and display it in a place that he looks at frequently as a reminder to think positively and stay focused on positive thoughts.

Variations of the activity

- This activity also works well in a group setting.
- This activity can also be completed using the individual's name or initials.

Discussion questions

- Why is it important to think positively?
- What are some things that you can do to stay focused on positive things?
- What are some words or phrases that are positive as well as meaningful to you?
- What happens when we start focusing on the negative instead of the positive?

- What are some signs or symptoms that you are thinking about or focusing on negative things instead of positive things?

- How can you turn your thinking around when it starts to go into a negative thought pattern?

- What is one new strategy that you can try to increase your focus on the positive?

- How are you going to use the Positive Word Art to remember to stay focused and think positively?

THESE ARE A FEW OF MY FAVORITE THINGS

Purpose of the activity

- To promote communication skills

- To develop positive self-concept

- To identify preferred items that can be used as incentives or reinforcers for the student

Materials needed

- Copies of the These are a Few of My Favorite Things Handout

- Pencils, pens, markers

Description of the activity

Explain to the group that today's activity is simply to find out about the individual's likes and some of his "favorite" things. Discuss with the individual the importance of being self-aware and expressing his likes and dislikes in a healthy manner. Tell the individual that it is also important for people who work with him to know about his favorite things so that these can be used as rewards and incentives when he displays good behavior or meets his goals. Provide the individual with a copy of the These are a Few of My Favorite Things Handout and writing supplies. Ask him to complete the handout and then share it with you. This can be kept to refer back to when it is time for the individual to earn a reward or an incentive.

Variations of the activity

- This activity also works well in groups. When complete, the participants can share their favorite things with a partner and then tell the group about each other's favorite things as a means of building communication skills and group relationships.

- This can also be a helpful handout to give to parents to use for rewards and incentives at home.

Discussion questions

- Tell me about the items and activities that you listed on your These are a Few of My Favorite Things Handout.

- Which item or activity would you be the most motivated to earn?

- Did everyone in the group list the same things for their favorite things? Why or why not?

- Are your favorite things the same now as they were a year ago?

- Why is it important to be self-aware?

- What are some healthy ways that you can tell others about your likes and dislikes?

- What surprised you about your partner's favorite things?

- What did you have in common with your partner's favorite things?

- What was different between your favorite things and your partner's favorite things?

- What is the best reward or incentive that you could receive?

- Were you able to easily list your favorite things or did you have to think about your responses? Explain.

These are a Few of My Favorite Things Handout

Favorite drink: . . . . Favorite chips:. . . . .

Favorite candy: . . . . Favorite food: . . . .

Favorite game: . . . . Favorite sport:. . . . .

Favorite friend: . . . . Favorite teacher: . . . .

Favorite subject: . . . . Favorite hobby: . . . .

Favorite movie: . . . . Favorite TV show:. . . . .

Favorite holiday: . . . . Favorite book:. . . . .

Favorite song: . . . . Favorite singer: . . . .

Favorite reward: . . . . Favorite art activity: . . . .

Favorite thing to do during free time: . . . .

Favorite things to do with my friends: . . . .

Favorite things to do at school: . . . .

Favorite things to do at home:. . . . .

POSITIVE THOUGHT SUNBURST ART

Purpose of the activity

- To develop positive thinking skills
- To encourage self-expression in a positive manner
- To promote positive social skills

Materials needed

- Paper
- Rulers
- Compass or small circular item (to trace for sunburst)
- Colored pencils, crayons
- Pens, pencils

Description of the activity

Begin the discussion with the students by talking about the sun. The sun is always warm and full of light that radiates to the planets around it. When we are standing in the sun, we can see because of the sun's light and feel warm because of the heat and warmth that the sun provides. Explain that positive thinking can be compared to the sun. As we keep ourselves "warm and full of light" with positive thinking, we are able to stay positive ourselves and radiate our light to those around us. Provide the individual with the needed supplies. Ask him to draw a circle in the middle of the paper and then use the ruler to draw lines radiating out from the circle to the edge of the paper. Ask the individual to color in the sunburst as desired using the colored pencils or crayons. When complete, ask him to use the pen to write his name in the center of the circle. Next, ask the individual to write positive thoughts and phrases in between the lines that are radiating out from the sunburst. These statements can be positive thoughts about the individual or positive thoughts about others. When he finishes, ask him to share the thoughts he wrote by reading them out loud and telling you about them.

Variations of the activity

- This activity can work well as part of a science unit on the sun and planets.
- This activity also works well as a group activity. Group members can create their own Positive Thought Sunburst Art as described above or, alternatively, create their own sunbursts and then pass them around so that the other group members can write positive thoughts about each individual on their artwork. Using this method with a group is a great way to build group unity as well as for the group members to develop social skills.
- This activity makes a great display for bulletin boards and group spaces. The heading "We are Bursting with Positive Thoughts" could be used.

Discussion questions

- How does the sun and the light it radiates compare to positive thinking?

- Does the sun warm only itself or does it warm others, too? How is this similar to positive thinking?

- When we think positively, it naturally spreads to others. Why do you think this is true?

- What are some reasons that we should think positively about ourselves?

- What are some reasons that we should think positively about others?

- Do you prefer to be around people who think positively and have good attitudes or people who think negatively and have bad attitudes? Why?

- How can you keep your thoughts focused on positive thoughts?

- What can you do to change the focus if you begin to think about negative things?

- Was it easier to write positive thoughts about yourself or others? Why or why not?

- (if using the group variation) How did you feel reading the positive thoughts that the other group members wrote about you?

- (if using the group variation) How did you feel writing the positive things about the other group members on their sunbursts?

- What are some ways that you can use your Positive Thought Sunburst Art to keep your thoughts focused on positive things?

- What is one new positive thought or strategy that you can use to promote positive thinking on a daily basis?

- What did you learn from this activity?

- What did you like about this activity?

- What was challenging about this activity?

HANDPRINT THANK-YOU NOTES

Purpose of the activity

- To express gratitude and thankfulness for others
- To develop positive social skills
- To promote positive thinking skills

Materials needed

- Colored paper (two pieces)
- Copies of the "Thank-You" Template Handout
- Paint
- Paint brushes
- Pens, colored pencils
- Envelopes
- Hole puncher
- Yarn, ribbon, or string
- Scissors

Description of the activity

Begin the discussion by talking about gratitude. Explain to the participant that no matter how "bad" things are, there is always something to be thankful for in our lives. Ask the participant to reflect on an individual who has made a difference in his life. This could be a parent, teacher, friend, sibling, or anyone else who is meaningful to the individual. Explain to the individual that it is important to let others know that they are appreciated and valued. Tell the individual that he will be creating a handmade thank-you note to give to the person who made a difference in his life. Provide him with the needed supplies. Begin by painting the individual's hand and having him make a painted handprint (facing downward) on one of the pieces of colored paper. Allow this to dry. When this is dry, ask the individual to write the following in a decorative manner around his handprint: "Hands down...you're the best around." Give him a copy of the "Thank-You" Template Handout and ask him to complete it with a meaningful message to the recipient. For younger children, assistance can be provided with writing the thank-you note. When the individual has finished the "Thank-You" Template, he can cut it out and glue it to the second piece of colored paper. Next, punch a hole in the top corner of both pieces of paper, tie them together with the yarn, string, or ribbon and place in the envelope for the individual to give to the chosen recipient.

Variations of the activity

- This activity is a good choice for Teacher Appreciation Week, Mother's Day, Father's Day, or Grandparents' Day.

Discussion questions

- What does it mean to be thankful or grateful?

- Do you believe that there is always something to be thankful for in our lives? Why or why not?

- What are some ways that we can show our gratitude to others and let others know that we appreciate them?

- Who has made a difference in your life?

- Does that person know how much you appreciate them and that you are grateful for his or her influence in your life?

- How can being grateful and appreciative of the good things in our lives influence our thinking? (The more we focus on positive things, the more positive we will be.)

- What are some ways that you may take for granted some of the good things in your life?

- What are some ways that you can become more thankful and aware of the good things in your life instead of taking them for granted?

- How did you choose the person to create your thank-you note for? Are there other people you could send one to?

- What did you think about this activity?

- Was there anything challenging about this activity? If so, what was it?

- What new strategy can you use to focus more on the positive and express more gratitude in your life?

- (at the next session) How did the recipient respond when you gave him or her the thank-you note? Was the experience a positive one for you?

"Thank-You" Template Handout

Dear . . . .

Thank you for . . . .

. . . .

. . . .

It means so much to me because . . . .

. . . .

. . . .

Thank you again for . . . .

. . . .

Sincerely,

. . . .

Date . . . .

PAINT CHIP REMINDER STRIPS

Purpose of the activity

- To develop coping skills and anger management skills
- To encourage positive thinking skills
- To promote self-awareness

Materials needed

- Paint chip strips in shades of blue and red (available at home improvement stores and paint stores)
- Hole puncher
- Yarn, string, or ribbon
- Pens or markers

Description of the activity

Ask the individual to think of some color associations for anger and calmness. Often, people may say "seeing red" to describe being angry, frustrated, or upset and associate the color red with anger. In contrast, the color blue is often associated with calmness, peace, and being cool. Provide the individual with a copy of the red tones paint strip. Ask the individual to identify some of his personal triggers and signs that he is becoming angry. Examples might be clenched fists or feeling hot. Discuss with the individual how his anger or frustration may then escalate. For example, he may get out of his seat, pace around, or stop completing his work. Finally, the anger may escalate to yelling, angry outbursts, or even aggression. Explain to the individual that it is important to be able to identify triggers for and symptoms of his anger so that it can be stopped before it escalates to a full outburst. On the red strip, ask the individual to list how his anger progresses, starting with how he feels when he first becomes upset or angry and then the things that happen as his anger continues to escalate. Ask the individual to write one symptom in each shade of red on the paint strip with the lightest color of red representing the start of his angry feelings and the darkest shade representing a full-blown angry outburst. When this is complete, provide the individual with the blue tone paint strip. Explain to him that it is important to learn to ways to calm down when he is feeling angry and to prevent his anger from escalating. Ask the individual to identify some strategies and techniques that he can use when he feels angry to stop the escalation of his anger. Examples might include asking for a break, walking away, going to a special cool down area, going to see his counselor, or taking deep breaths. Ask the individual to list a different anger management strategy in each shade of blue on the blue paint strip. He can also decorate his strip if desired. When complete, punch a hole in the top of the strip and allow the individual to choose a piece of yarn, ribbon, or string to tie on his Paint Chip Reminder Strips. These can be used as bookmarks or the individual can keep them with him in a folder at his desk to refer to when he becomes angry.

Variations of the activity

- This activity works well with lots of therapeutic or character education concepts. For example, the participant could create Paint Chip Reminder Strips for positive thoughts, classroom rules and expectations, and social skills reminders.

- These can also be a fun gift to create for others by listing positive things about the person and then tying with a pretty ribbon to create a bookmark.

Discussion questions

- What is a color that is associated with anger?

- What is a color that is associated with calmness and peace?

- What are some signs that you may be getting angry, upset, or frustrated?

- What are some changes that you feel in your body when you get angry, frustrated, or upset? Examples might be clenched fists, gritted teeth, and feeling hot.

- What happens if your anger continues to escalate?

- What are some strategies that you can use when you first start feeling upset or angry to prevent your anger from escalating?

- What anger management strategies have worked for you in the past?

- What are some situations that may trigger your anger?

- What are some strategies and techniques that you can list on your Paint Chip Reminder Strip to refer to when you are beginning to feel angry or upset?

- Where can you keep your Paint Strip Reminder Strips so that you can get to them easily and frequently be reminded of your strategies?

- What is one new strategy that you can try for anger management?

POSITIVE THOUGHT BUCKET

Purpose of the activity

- To encourage positive thinking
- To provide a visual reminder of positive thoughts
- To promote positive self-concept

Materials needed

- Small flower pot
- Large popsicle/craft sticks
- Paint
- Paint brushes
- Sharpie markers

Description of the activity

Ask each individual to identify some areas where they struggle with maintaining positive thoughts. Assist each individual with developing positive thoughts and affirmations for each of these areas. Explain that the activity will be to create a Positive Thought Bucket with the affirmation statements so that these can be frequently referred to. Provide the individual with the materials. Ask the individual to paint his flower pot which will be the Positive Thought Bucket in any way he wishes. When complete, allow to dry. While it is drying, ask him to list a positive affirmation on each of the popsicle or craft sticks. When complete, ask him to place his popsicle or craft sticks inside the painted flower pot (Positive Thought Bucket). Discuss with the individual ways to use the bucket each day. Examples might include pulling out a positive thought stick each morning or right before bed, pulling out a stick any time a negative thought comes into his head, etc.

Variation of the activity

- Make a Positive Thought Garden: this activity can be great in groups. Follow directions as above. Each individual's bucket can remain in the group meeting space. At the beginning of each group session, each member can pull a positive thought stick from his bucket and read it aloud to the group.

Discussion questions

- What are some negative thoughts that you struggle with at times?

- What are some positive statements that you can use to contradict the negative thoughts?

- Why is it important to focus on the positive instead of the negative?

- What strategies can you use to "change your thoughts" when they tend toward the negative?

- What are some ways that you can keep focused on the positives in your life?

- How can you use your Positive Thought Bucket to encourage more positive thinking in your life?

MUSICAL CHAIRS ART

Purpose of the activity

- To promote social skills
- To encourage group unity and cohesiveness
- To provide opportunities for creativity

Materials needed

- Paper (one sheet per group member)
- Markers or colored pencils (one color per group member)
- Table with chairs or group of desks arranged in a circle
- CD and CD player or other method of playing music

Description of the activity

Ask the participants if they have ever played musical chairs before, and explain that the group will be playing a variation of this game. Each person will select one color to use throughout the entire activity. Each group member will be given a piece of paper at his seat. Next, the group leader will begin playing music. As long as the music is playing, the participants will draw using their chosen color on their paper. When the group leader stops the music, everyone will stop drawing and move one seat to the right. When the group leader starts the music again, the group members will add to the drawing at their new seat using their chosen color. This process will continue until the group members have rotated back around to their original seats. At the conclusion of the activity, each group member will have a drawing that has all the colors representing each of the group members and the group as a whole.

Variations of the activity

- This activity can also be used with other forms of art media such as paint, collage, mosaic, etc.
- It could also be completed by assigning an object to each participant. For example, one participant could be assigned houses, another flowers, another animals. Each person could draw their object on their own drawing during the musical rotations.
- It could also be used for writing group poems or short stories. Each participant could start a poem or story to which the other members would add during the musical rotations.
- These make a great display in the group area with the heading "The Colors of Us."

Discussion questions

- What was your favorite thing about this activity?

- What was challenging about this activity?

- What was it like to have to leave your original drawing without completing it and then have others add to it?

- How did you decide what to add to the other group members' drawings?

- What did you think of your original drawing when you got back to your seat? Were you surprised at how your drawing turned out?

- What did you notice about each of the completed drawings? (One thing might be that each drawing included all of the colors so each group member was represented in each drawing.)

- How did each drawing represent each group member individually as well as the group as a whole?

- What would change about the drawings if you removed some of the colors? Would the drawings be as colorful and beautiful? What if the drawing only had one color?

- How did you use your social skills as you were completing this activity with the other group members?

HELPING HANDS MITTEN FRIEND

Purpose of the activity

- To develop positive coping skills
- To encourage positive thinking skills
- To promote creativity and self-expression

Materials needed

- Mittens (one for each group member—bright colors if possible)
- Fabric glue
- Tacky glue
- Filler for stuffing the mitten
- Small eyes or buttons (found in the craft section at stores)
- Assorted colors of small buttons or pom poms (for nose)
- Pipe cleaners or small piece of felt (cut in the shape of a mouth)

Description of the activity

Begin by discussing coping skills with the individual. There are many different ways to cope with stress and difficult situations. Individuals might talk to a trusted friend, keep a journal, exercise, have some quiet time, etc. For little children, a security object such as a blanket or teddy bear can also promote coping skills. Explain to the individual that he is going to create a Helping Hands Mitten Friend to remind him to use his positive coping skills whenever he feels stressed, worried, upset, or angry. Allow the individual to select a mitten to create his Helping Hands Mitten Friend. Provide the individual with the filler and ask him to stuff the filling inside the mitten until it is full. Seal the glove closed using the fabric glue and allow it time to dry. Next, provide the individual with the buttons, felt, and pom poms and ask him to create a face on his mitten using the materials. It works best to put the mouth at the bottom of the glove and the eyes at the top near the fingers, because then the Helping Hands Mitten Friend can stand on its own or be propped on something (it will not prop or stand as well on the fingers end of the mitten). When the individual has arranged the face as desired on his Helping Hands Mitten Friend, glue the pieces of the face on as desired and allow time for it to dry. Discuss with the individual ways that his Helping Hands Mitten Friend can remind him of his coping skills. This activity works well with lower elementary students.

Variations of the activity

- This activity could also be completed with colorful socks (Coping Skills Caterpillar).

Discussion questions

- What are coping skills?

- What are some situations or times in your life when you will need to use your coping skills?

- What are some positive coping skills that you can use in your life when you feel stressed, worried, or upset?

- Do you have a favorite stuffed animal or blanket? How does this help you to cope? (Does it calm you at night if you are by yourself?)

- How can the Helping Hands Mitten Friend remind you to use your positive coping skills?

- Where will you keep your Helping Hands Mitten Friend so that it can be a frequent reminder to you to use your positive coping skills?

- Tell me about a time when you used coping skills to deal with a stressful situation in a positive and healthy way.

- What is one new positive coping skill that you can try?

INSIDE MY HEAD SILHOUETTE

Purpose of the activity

- To promote healthy self-expression and creativity
- To develop communication skills
- To express thoughts and feelings in a positive manner

Materials needed

- Flashlight
- Large piece of paper or poster-board
- Tape
- Pencil
- Markers
- Magazines and other materials for a collage
- Scissors
- Glue

Description of the activity

Explain to the individual that he is going to create an Inside My Head Silhouette. Start by taping the piece of paper to the wall in a dark room. Place the flashlight on a table and shine the light toward the paper. Next, ask the individual to sit on a stool or chair in between the paper and the flashlight. Adjust the height of the paper (if needed) so that the shadow of the individual's profile appears on the paper. Trace the outline of the individual's profile onto the paper using the pencil. Take the piece of paper down from the wall and trace over the pencil outline with a black marker. After this is complete, discuss with the individual the expression "inside my head." Ask him to identify some of the things that have been going on in his head. What does he find himself thinking about frequently? Does he ever get certain thoughts stuck in his head? What are his likes and dislikes? Ask him to create a collage of what is going on inside his head by selecting images to glue onto the inside of his silhouette representing the things that are "inside his head." The markers can also be used to write phrases or words, or draw pictures on the silhouette. When complete, discuss the images that the individual selected and what each image represents to him.

Variations of the activity

- If desired, the silhouette can be cut out and pasted onto a piece of black paper to have the look of a true silhouette.
- This activity is great for groups. Group member can introduce themselves to the group using their Inside My Head Silhouette to talk about what is going on inside their head.
- This activity also makes a great display using the heading "What's Going on Inside Our Heads."

Discussion questions

- What does the expression "inside my head" mean?

- What are some of the things that are "inside your head" right now?

- Tell me about the images, words, or phrases that you included on your Inside My Head Silhouette.

- How do you feel about your completed Inside My Head Silhouette? Is it a true reflection of you and what's inside your head? Why or why not?

- What do you think your Inside My Head Silhouette might say about you to someone who doesn't know you?

- Are there any recurring images or words on your Inside My Head Silhouette? If so, what are they?

- What did you enjoy about creating your Inside My Head Silhouette?

- What was challenging about creating your Inside My Head Silhouette?

- Did you learn anything about yourself or gain any self-awareness through creating and discussing your Inside My Head Silhouette? If so, what was it?

WEATHER EMOTION PAPER PLATE

Purpose of the activity

- To learn about and understand various feelings
- To identify healthy ways to express feelings
- To encourage positive coping skills

Materials needed

- Two paper plates per participant
- Scissors
- Glue
- Construction paper (yellow, orange, blue, gray, black)
- Paint
- Paint brushes
- Yarn
- Hole puncher
- Colored pencils, markers, crayons

Description of the activity

Begin by discussing some of the different types of weather with the participant. Discuss with him that various feelings and moods are often associated with different types of weather. For example, sunny days are often associated with happiness. Expressions such as "bright, sunshiny day" and "clear skies ahead" are frequently used to denote the happiness that is linked to sunny weather. Rainy days can be associated with sadness. Expressions such as "rainy, dreary day" and "rain, rain, go away, come again another day" are frequently used to denote the sadness that can be associated with rainy days. Stormy days with lightning and thunder are often associated with anger. Expressions such as "angry skies" and "powerful storms" are used to denote the anger that can be linked to strong thunderstorms.

Explain to the participant that he is going to create some Weather Emotion Paper Plates to learn more about his feelings and emotions and how to deal with them. Provide him with the necessary supplies. Ask him to cut the paper plates in half and paint one half of a plate yellow (to denote the sun), one half of a plate blue (to denote the rain), and one half of a plate black (to denote stormy weather). The remaining plate half could be saved for use in another activity or discarded. While the paint is drying, cut the construction paper into strips (the yellow and orange strips go with the sun plate, the blue and gray strips go with the rain plate, and the black and gray strips go with the stormy plate). Ask the individual to write some other words or phrases for the feeling on one side of the strip (use a white pencil or crayon for it to show up on the black construction paper). For example, happiness can also be associated with joy, ease, pleasure, etc. Sadness could be associated with crying, depression, feeling down, etc. Anger could be associated with rage, aggression, feeling mad, etc. When this is complete, ask the individual to turn the strips over and write some ways to handle each of the feelings. For example, some ways to cope with happiness might be to enjoy it and share it with others. Some ways to cope with sadness might be to talk to a friend or participate in a fun activity. Some ways to cope with anger might be to ask for a cool down time or use deep breathing. When the paint on the paper plate halves is dry, the participant can create a face on each one by either drawing or cutting facial shapes out of the leftover construction paper and gluing them on the plate. He could also cut triangles or zigzags to glue to the top of the plate to represent the sun's ray or lightning bolts during a storm. Next, glue the strips that each participant wrote on to the bottom of the paper plate so that they hang down. Use the hole puncher to punch a hole in the top center of the plate, place yarn in the hole, and hang it in a desired location.

Variations of the activity

- The Weather Emotion Paper Plates activity works well with groups. It is a great way to help younger children understand feelings and emotions. It could also be incorporated into a science unit on the weather.

- The plates make a great display using the heading "Our Weather Report on Feelings."

- The participant can also give a "weather report" on his feelings at the beginning of sessions.

Discussion questions

- What are some different types of weather? What are some expressions and feelings associated with different types of weather?

- What are some other words and phrases to describe feeling happy?

- What are some ways to handle happiness?

- What are some other words and phrases to describe feeling sad?

- What are some ways to cope when you feel sad?

- What are some other words and phrases to describe feeling angry?

- What are some ways to cope with anger?

- Why is it important to be able to name and understand our feelings?

- What did you learn from completing this activity?

HIGH FIVES FOR MY FRIENDS

(For a similar icebreaker activity refer to page 28.)

Purpose of the activity

- To develop positive social skills
- To encourage positive thinking
- To promote healthy relationship and friendships

Materials needed

- Construction paper
- Scissors
- Markers, pencils, pens
- Hole puncher
- Yarn or ribbon

Description of the activity

Begin by asking the participant if he has ever received a "high five." A high five is a hand gesture used to say "good job" or "I am proud of you." Explain to the participant that he is going to create a lasting "high five" to give to a friend. Ask the individual to trace his hand and then use the scissors to cut the handprint out. Ask him to think of a friend in his life who means a lot to him. Ask him to think of five positive things about the friend and to write these on each of the fingers on the handprint. Next, ask him to use the markers to write the friend's name on the palm part of the hand and then decorate the handprint. The participant can punch a hole underneath the friend's name and tie with yarn or ribbon if desired. Allow the individual to take the handprint to give to his friend.

Variations of the activity

- This activity also makes a great gift for family members, especially for Mother's Day or Father's Day.
- The activity also works well for groups. Each member can create a High Five to give to each of the other group members. Holes can be punched at the bottom of each handprint, and all the handprints can be tied together using the yarn or ribbon. Each group member then has all of his High Fives together in one place as a keepsake of positive thoughts from the other group members.

- From time to time the group leader can also make the participants point out positive things or note the accomplishments of other group members.

Discussion questions

- What is a high five?
- What does it mean when someone says "Give me a high five?"
- How does it feel to receive a high five from someone when you have done something positive?
- Which friend in your life means so much to you that you would like to give him or her a lasting high five?
- What are some positive traits and qualities about your friend?
- What are things that your friend has accomplished?
- How do you think your friend will feel to receive the High Fives for My Friends handprint that you created for him?
- Why is it important to tell others that we appreciate them and to point out their positive qualities?
- How can you continue to use the idea of "giving high fives to others" in your life?
- What are some additional ways to show others how much you appreciate them or to say positive things to them?

If the group version is used:

- How did it feel to write all of the positive things about the other group members on your High Fives for My Friends and then give it to them?
- How did it feel to receive the High Fives for My Friends from all of the other group members with positive statements about you written on them?
- Did giving and receiving the High Fives for My Friends bring about any changes in the group? If so, what?
- What did you like about creating the High Fives for My Friends?
- What was challenging about giving or receiving the High Fives for My Friends?
- What did you learn from creating the High Fives for My Friends?

MEANINGFUL MONOGRAM

Purpose of the activity

- To promote positive self-concept

- To encourage creativity and self-expression

- To gain information and insight about the individual

Materials needed

- Drawing paper

- Colored pencils, pens, markers

- Examples of monograms in various styles (one initial, three initials, name, etc.) and with various types of lettering (script, block, etc.)

Description of the activity

Monograms have been used for many years to indicate ownership and provide a way to identify the individual or family. Explain to the participant that he is going to create a Meaningful Monogram. Show the participant examples of the various types of monograms and ask him to select the style and type of lettering to use for his Meaningful Monogram. Ask him to write the desired monogram in the chosen style and lettering on his paper. Next, ask him to think of some personal traits and characteristics that are unique to him. Ask him to think of some symbols or small drawings to reflect these individual characteristics and then draw them around his monogram in an artistic manner of his choice. For example, a dog lover might draw a dog, individuals who enjoy exercise might draw a bicycle or a running shoe, those who like to read might draw a book, and those who enjoy music might draw a music note. The possibilities are endless. After the individual has finished the drawing, he can add color and design to the monogram using the art supplies. Ask the individual to tell you about his monogram when complete.

Variations of the activity

- This activity works well in groups. Group members can share their Meaningful Monograms with the group when complete, helping to build communication skills and unity within the group. Older children and teenagers seem to enjoy this activity.

- These make a really nice display when mounted on construction paper in a coordinating color. The heading "Our Meaningful Monograms" can be used.

- The Meaningful Monogram can also be created as a gift. The participant can create a Meaningful Monogram about his family (using the last name) or one of his parents and give it as a gift. They make great gifts for Grandparent's Day, Mother's Day, Father's Day, or birthdays.

Discussion questions

- What is a monogram?
- What is the purpose of a monogram?
- Tell me about your Meaningful Monogram that you created.
- How did you select what to include on your Meaningful Monogram?
- What do you think your Meaningful Monogram says about you?
- What did you enjoy about creating your Meaningful Monogram?
- What was challenging about creating it?

If using the group version:

- What did you learn about the other group members through their Meaningful Monograms? Were you surprised by anything on someone's Meaningful Monogram?
- Were all of the Meaningful Monograms alike? Why or why not?
- Would it have been as fun or interesting to create the Meaningful Monograms if everyone's monogram had to look alike?
- Why is it important to share details about ourselves with others? Why is it important to listen and pay attention when others share details about themselves with us?

POSITIVE POM POM LETTERS

Purpose of the activity

- To develop perseverance and patience
- To promote positive self-concept
- To build skills in following directions

Materials needed

- Canvas or heavy-weight paper
- Pencil, black marker
- Tacky glue
- Pom poms in assorted colors and sizes (found in the craft section at stores)

Description of the activity

Explain to the individual that the activity will take some time and patience but the end result will be worth it. Using the pencil write the first letter of the individual's name on the canvas or heavy-weight paper. The letter can be written in script, block, or any other format the individual chooses. Next, trace over the letter in the black marker to make it easier to see and follow. Ask the individual to work in one section at a time by first putting some of the tacky glue on a small section of the letter and then placing the pom poms on top of the glue. Tweezers can be used to pick up and place the pom poms if desired. The individual can choose to use all of the same color or size pom poms or use a variety of color and size pom poms to create the desired effect. Ask the individual to repeat the above process until the letter is completely covered in pom poms. The Positive Pom Pom Letters make a great display for the individual to take home for his room.

Variations of the activity

- This is a good activity for groups. While it works well for each group member to create a letter using his first initial as described above, group unity and relationships can also be built up by working together to create a word. Each member creates one letter of the word. For example, if the word "hope" is chosen, then one member creates the "H," one member creates the "o," and so on. These can then be displayed in the group meeting space.

Discussion questions

- What traits did it require for you to complete this activity?

- What would the letter have looked like if you had only completed one small section with pom poms and then stopped?

- Why is it important to complete things that we start and exhibit perseverance in our lives?

- What did your Positive Pom Pom Letter look like when it was complete? Was it worth all of the effort to complete it?

- What did you like about this activity?

- What was challenging about this activity?

- Where will you display your Positive Pom Pom Letter? What are some things that you will be reminded of when you look at it?

If using the group version:

- What is special about this word that the group chose to create using Positive Pom Pom Letters?

- How long would it have taken one person to spell out the word by themselves in pom pom letters? How long did it take with the group working together and each person creating one of the letters? Which way do you think is the better choice?

- How does the word reflect each person in the group?

THUMBPRINT TREE

Purpose of the activity

- To build group unity and relationships
- To provide a visual image of the group for the group meeting space
- To provide a means for new group members to gain a sense of belonging and unity with the group

Materials needed

- Copies of the Thumbprint Tree Handout or a large drawing of a tree with branches (the group can work together to create the tree on a large piece of paper if desired)
- Ink pad

Description of the activity

Begin by explaining to the group that they are going to create a Thumbprint Tree. If the group is going to draw and paint the tree themselves, allow them to do so. When complete, ask each group member to select a branch. Using the ink pad, ask the group members to put their thumbs in the ink and then press them down on the chosen tree branches as desired. If a larger tree was created, the individual may be able to put multiple thumbprints on his tree branch.

If using the Thumbprint Tree Handout, allow each individual to select a branch and then place his thumb in the stamp pad and make a thumbprint on the chosen branch. The Thumbprint Tree can be kept in the group meeting space. If new members are added to the group, then they can add their thumbprint to the tree on their first day to create a sense of belonging and unity with the existing group members.

Variations of the activity

- Handprints could also be used instead of thumbprints if a larger tree is created by the group.
- This is also a great project for a family to create. The family can create a family tree using thumbprints. Each family member can write his or her name underneath his or her thumbprint. The tree can be painted with watercolors or colored with markers or colored pencils. This makes a great gift for family members.

Discussion questions

- How does the Thumbprint Tree represent the group as a whole?
- How is each individual person represented on the tree?
- Are all of the thumbprints exactly alike? Why or why not?

- How can we welcome new members to our group?
- Why is it important to help others feel that they belong?
- What are some of the positive things about getting a new member in our group?
- What are some of the challenges about getting a new member in our group?
- What did you like about this activity?
- What did you learn from this activity?

Thumbprint Tree Handout

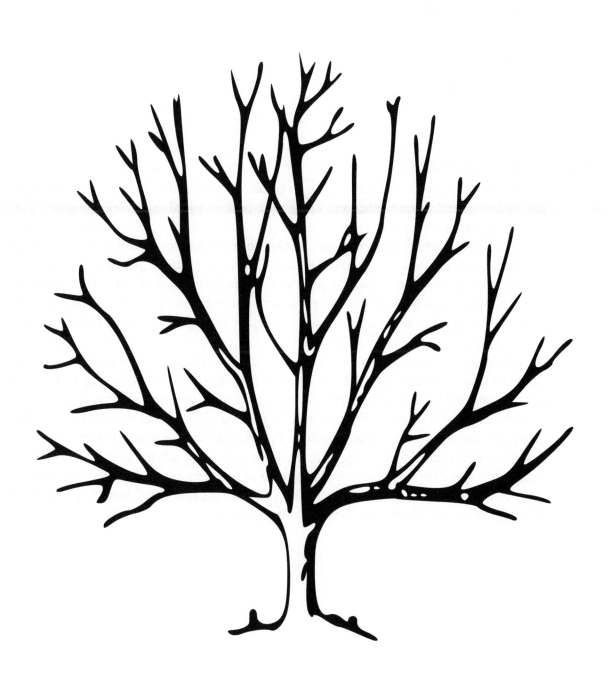

KINDNESS CHAIN

Purpose of the activity

- To encourage kindness and other positive behaviors
- To build group unity and relationship among group members
- To develop positive social skills

Materials needed

- Construction paper
- Scissors
- Markers
- Stapler, staples
- Thumbtack

Description of the activity

Explain to the group that they are going to be able to help each other earn a group party just by being kind to each other and using their positive social skills. Tell the group that you (the group leader) will be watching everyone closely. Each time you notice someone doing something kind for someone else or using their positive social skills in a challenging situation, you will add a link to the Kindness Chain. When the Kindness Chain reaches the floor, the group will be allowed a party of their choice to celebrate all of their kindness and positive social skills. Start the group out with one chain link (one strip of construction paper stapled together at the ends to form a circle) for using good listening skills while you told them about the activity. For each chain link, cut a strip of construction paper and then circle it around the previous link in the chain and staple. Using the thumbtack, attach the Kindness Chain to the top of a bulletin board or near the top of a wall. During each group meeting, try to find at least two acts of kindness by two different members to add to the Kindness Chain. When you notice an act of kindness or positive behavior, stop and tell the group that you will be adding to the chain. Tell them which group member you observed doing something kind. Cut a strip of construction paper and ask the group member who exhibited the kind behavior to come and write his or her name or initials on the construction paper and decorate as desired. When complete, add it to the Kindness Chain. Continue until the chain reaches the floor, and celebrate with a group party.

Variations of the activity

- This activity can also be used to promote a specific behavior. Instead of kindness or positive social skills in general, you may choose to focus on a specific behavior that needs to be cultivated within your group. Examples might include anger management skills, conflict resolution skills, or positive thinking skills. If anger management is the chosen focus area, then each time you see a group member exhibit positive anger management skills, you add a link to the chain.

- This activity can also be used for goal setting with individuals. Assist the individual in a breaking his goal down into a series of steps. Each time the individual completes a step toward his goal, a link can be added to his chain as a visual reminder of his progress.

Discussion questions

- What are some examples of acts of kindness and ways to show kindness to others?
- What are some examples of positive social skills?
- How does the Kindness Chain work?
- How can links be added to the Kindness Chain?
- How long will it take for the Kindness Chain to reach the floor if only one group member is exhibiting kindness to others or positive social skills?
- How long will it take if everyone is exhibiting acts of kindness and positive social skills?
- Do you prefer to be around people who are kind? Why or why not?
- If everyone prefers kind people, then why is hard to be kind to others?
- What is one new act of kindness that you can start exhibiting to your friends and family?

WORRY WORMS

Purpose of the activity

- To identify worries and other negative thoughts
- To encourage positive coping skills
- To promote healthy self-expression

Materials needed

- Small smooth sticks (gathered from outside)
- Assorted colors of pipe cleaners
- Small pom pom for head
- Small eyes (found in the craft section at stores)
- Tacky glue
- Small strips of paper
- Pencil

Description of the activity

Begin by asking the individual what it means to worry. When we get a worry in our head, it often seems to be all we can think about and it gets "stuck." The worry thoughts keep going around and around in our heads, constantly moving. Explain that worms are constantly on the move, too…just like the worry thoughts. Tell the individual that today he is going to create a Worry Worm. Whenever he feels a worry thought, he can give it to the worm and the worm will take the worry thought with it. Provide the participant with the strips of paper and pencil. Ask him to write some of his worries that get stuck in his head on the strips of paper. Next, he can fold the strips of paper up and set them aside while he creates his Worry Worm. Provide the individual with the remaining supplies. Ask him to select two colors of pipe cleaners. Assist him in twisting the pipe cleaners around the stick. The pipe cleaners should be tight enough that they will not come off the stick but loose enough to allow for the small strips of paper to be inserted in between the pipe cleaners. When this is complete, assist the individual in attaching the pom pom to serve as the head to the end of the stick using the tacky glue. Next, attach the small eyes to the pom pom head on the front of the stick using the tacky glue. If needed, the pipe cleaners can also be glued to the stick at the ends to help them stay attached. After the worm is finished, ask the individual to stick the strips of paper with his worries written on them in between the pipe cleaners on the worm. Once the individual gives the strips of paper to the worm, the worm will carry them away and the individual does not have to think about them anymore. The individual can take the worry worm and some of the strips of paper with him after the session and each time he has a worry thought, he can write it on the paper and give it to the Worry Worm.

Variations of the activity

- This is also a good activity for groups and works well with elementary age children.

- This activity can also be used for other types of thoughts, such as negative thoughts and angry thoughts.

- A great continuation of this activity is to create a Positive Thoughts Flower. For each worry thought, replacement thoughts can be developed. See the Positive Thoughts Flower activity for more details.

Discussion questions

- What does it mean to worry?

- How do you feel when you worry?

- Do you ever get worry thoughts "stuck" in your head? How do you handle this?

- What are some of the worries that you wrote on your strips of paper?

- Why is it important to get worries out of your head and give them to the Worry Worm to carry away?

- After you write down your worries and give them to your Worry Worm, what are some things that you can do to make sure that you don't start worrying about the same things again?

- When you worry about things, are you solving the problem or doing anything positive about the things that you are worried about?

- How will your Worry Worm serve as a visual symbol or reminder to let go of your worries?

- What is one new strategy that you can use when you start to worry?

- What did you like about creating the Worry Worm?

- What did you learn from this activity?

- Where will you keep your Worry Worm so that you can remember to give your worry thoughts to it?

POSITIVE THOUGHTS FLOWER

Purpose of the activity

- To develop positive thinking skills
- To promote coping skills
- To encourage replacement thoughts for worries and other negative thought patterns

Materials needed

- Copies of the Positive Thoughts Flower Handout
- Scissors
- Crayons, colored pencils
- Pens, pencils
- Craft or popsicle sticks (found in the craft section at stores)
- Glue

Description of the activity

The Positive Thoughts Flower is a great follow-up activity to the Worry Worm activity (see previous activity). Explain to the participant that while it is important to get worries and other negative thoughts out of our minds, it is also important to fill our minds with positive thoughts. We need positive thoughts to "replace" the worries and negative thoughts that the Worry Worm took for us. Ask the participant to think about some of the worry thoughts that he wrote on his strips of paper while completing the Worry Worm activity. Assist him in developing positive thoughts to "replace" each of the worries. For example, if one of his worries was "No one likes me," then a replacement thought might be "I make friends easily and lots of people like me." Provide the participant with the needed supplies. Ask him to write his name in the center of the flower template and then write one of the positive replacement thoughts in each of the petals of the flower. Next, he can color and decorate the flower as he chooses. When this is complete, the flower can be cut out and the stem can be glued to the craft stick in order to make it more sturdy.

Variations of the activity

- This activity works well in groups. A Garden of Positive Thought Flowers can be created as a display in the room. Group members can read aloud some of the positive statements on their flowers at the beginning or end of each group session to emphasize the importance of positive self-talk.

- For an extension of the activity, a small flower pot can be purchased and painted for the participant to keep the Worry Worm (from the previous activity) and the Positive Thoughts Flower in after the sessions. Consider having the participant cut out a few blank flower templates as well. When the individual is at home and has a new worry thought that he gives to the Worry Worm, he can immediately develop a positive replacement thought to write on one of the blank flower templates. By keeping everything in the small flower pot, the participant will have all of the supplies together and easily accessible when he has a worry thought.

Discussion questions

- What does it mean to think positively?

- What is a positive thought to "replace" one of your worry thoughts?

- Why is it important to think positively?

- How can the Worry Worm and Positive Thoughts Flower help you remember to stop thinking about your worry thoughts and start thinking about your positive replacement thoughts?

- How does the statement "we get more of what we focus on" apply to the thoughts we think?

- What would happen if you just gave your worry thoughts to your Worry Worm, but didn't develop any positive replacement thoughts? Do you think the worry thoughts might eventually come back?

- Who gets to decide the thoughts you will think and focus on in your mind?

- What is one new strategy that you can use to develop more positive thinking in your life?

- How will your Positive Thoughts Flower help you remember to think positively?

- What did you like about creating the Positive Thoughts Flower?

- What did you learn from creating the Positive Thoughts Flower?

Positive Thoughts Flower Handout

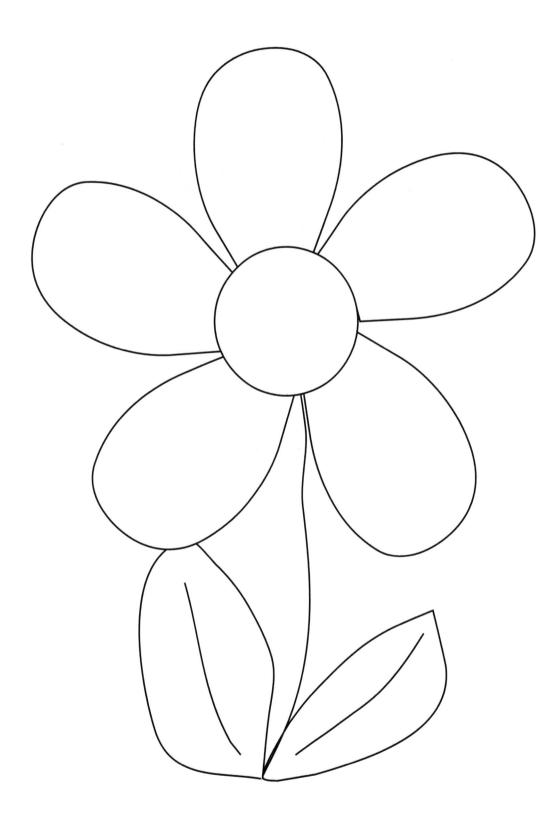

SHINY, HAPPY PEOPLE

Purpose of the activity

- To identify and understand feelings and emotions (especially happiness)
- To promote creativity and self-expression
- To develop coping skills and positive thinking skills

Materials needed

- Aluminum foil
- Cardboard (from leftover boxes)
- Paint
- Paint brushes

Description of the activity

Discuss happiness with the participant. Explain that sometimes a person may feel sad or angry for so long he does not understand happiness or how to feel happy. Explain that it is important to recognize when we are happy, to take time to enjoy ourselves, and to take care of ourselves. Tell the participant that he is going to create a self-portrait of himself when he is happy. The self-portrait will be completed on the aluminum foil. It is fun to paint on aluminum foil and the shiny background makes the bright colors of the paint really stand out. Begin by covering the cardboard with the aluminum foil. Provide the participant with paint and brushes and ask him to create a self-portrait of himself when he is happy on the aluminum foil-covered cardboard. While completing the activity, discuss happiness, positive leisure activities, self-care strategies, and ways to enjoy feeling happy.

Variations of the activity

- This activity works well for groups. The self-portraits make a great display using the heading "Shiny Happy People."
- The participants could also paint an image or design that makes them feel happy instead of self-portraits.

Discussion questions

- What does it mean to be happy?
- What is your definition of happiness?
- How would someone know if you were happy?
- Does it feel strange to be happy if you have been sad or angry for a long time?
- What are some positive ways to handle the feeling of happiness?

- What are some activities that you enjoy doing when you have free time?

- What does it mean to take care of yourself or use self-care strategies?

- Why it is important to take care of ourselves?

- How can you share the feeling of being happy with others when you are happy?

- What are some ways that you can make more time for things you enjoy in your life and for using your self-care strategies?

- Tell me about your Shiny, Happy People self-portrait.

- Where will you display your Shiny, Happy People self-portrait to remind you that it is okay to feel happy and to take care of yourself in healthy ways?

- What did you enjoy about creating your self-portrait?

- What was challenging about creating your self-portrait?

- What did you learn from this activity?

BAD HAIR DAY ART

Purpose of the activity

- To identify triggers or setting factors that may influence the participant to have a "bad day"
- To promote positive coping skills
- To develop an understanding and awareness of self and feelings

Materials needed

- Copies of the Bad Hair Day Art Handouts
- Copies of the Examples of Lines Handout
- Pens, markers, colored pencils
- Ruler

Description of the activity

Begin by asking the participant if he has ever heard someone say, "I'm having a bad hair day." While this phrase is usually used to describe someone who is literally having a day when their hair does not look great, it can often imply that a person's whole day is not going well because their hair does not look the way they like it to look. For example, the day may start out bad because of the "bad hair" and then continue to get worse due to the bad mood that the person may be in because of the "bad hair." Explain to the participant that he is going to create a Bad Hair Day Art project while discussing some of the factors in his life that may cause him to have a "bad hair day," and how to cope with days that are not so great. Provide the participant with the handouts, markers, colored pencils, and ruler. Ask him to create a drawing of someone who is having a "bad hair day" using a variety of the different lines (see the Examples of Lines Handout) and patterns on the Bad Hair Day Art Handout. The participant may choose to add color to his Bad Hair Day Art after adding the various lines and patterns. When complete, discuss some of the factors and events that may trigger him to have a "bad hair day" or just a "bad day," as well as positive ways to cope with days that are not so great. After the individual has completed his Bad Hair Day Art project provide him with the Bad Hair Day Art Reflection Handout. Give him time to complete this and then discuss his responses. This could be completed in a second session if needed.

Variations of the activity

- This activity also works well with groups.
- The Bad Hair Day Art projects make a great display using the heading "We're having a Bad Hair Day!"

Discussion questions

- What is a "bad hair day?"

- Have you ever had a "bad hair day?" How did you feel on your "bad hair day?"

- Have you ever experienced a day when one "bad" thing happened and then everything else seemed to go wrong too? What was this day like for you?

- What are some things that might happen to trigger you to have a "bad" day?

- What does a "bad" day look and feel like for you?

- What are some positive ways to cope with a "bad hair day" kind of day?

- If something happens that upsets you, how can you turn your day around so that your whole day doesn't turn into a "bad" day?

- What are some of the types of lines and patterns you see on your Bad Hair Day Art?

- Are all of your lines going in the same direction or are the lines going in many different directions on your Bad Hair Day Art? (Discuss how sometimes a "bad" day may start when a person feels pulled in too many different directions.)

- Are some of the lines on your Bad Hair Day Art completely straight and rigid? (Discuss how sometimes a person may have a "bad" day when there is no flexibility and everything is rigid.)

- Do some of your lines and patterns have circles or designs that go around and around on your Bad Hair Day Art? (Discuss how sometimes a person may have a "bad" day when everything seems to be going in circles and they cannot seem to get out of the circle.)

- Do any of your lines have sharp ups and downs or zig zags on your Bad Hair Day Art? (Discuss how sometimes a person may have a "bad" day because their mood is constantly up and then down.)

- Are there any patterns on your Bad Hair Day Art? (Discuss how sometimes a "bad" day can occur when we exhibit the same patterns of behavior instead of trying new strategies and behaviors.)

- What are some positive coping skills that could be used to address each of the different types of "bad" days that a person might experience?

- What is one new coping strategy that you will try when you have a day that is not so great to try to "turn your day around" in a positive way?

- Where can you display your Bad Hair Day Art to remind yourself to handle "bad" days in a positive manner?

- What did you like about this activity?

- What was challenging about this activity?

- What did you learn from creating the Bad Hair Day Art?

This adaptation of content from the March 1997 issue of *Arts & Activities* magazine appears with permission from the publisher (www.artsandactivities.com).

Examples of Lines Handout

Straight line:

_____

Dotted line:

· ·

Dashed line:

– –

Bold line:

_____

Zig zag line:

VVVVVVVVVVVVVVVVVVVVVVVVVVVVVVVVVVVVVVVVVVVVVVVV

Wavy line:

~~~~~~~~~~~~~~~~~~~~~~~~~~~~~~~~~~~~~~

Curved line:

Bad Hair Day Art Handout

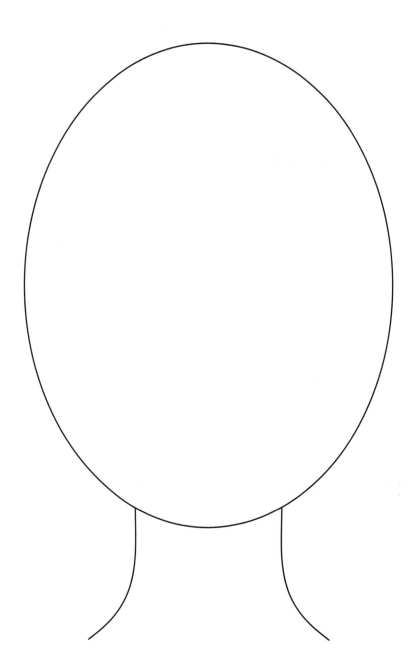

Use lines and patterns to create a "bad hair day" and face on the image above.

Bad Hair Day
Art Reflection Handout

A "bad hair day" feels like: . . . .

. . . .

When I have a "bad hair day," I will: . . . .

. . . .

I know it is going to be a "bad hair day" when: . . . .

. . . .

These are the patterns and lines I see in my Bad Hair Day Art:

. . . .

My art represents a "bad hair day" because: . . . .

I cope with a "bad hair day" by: . . . .

A "bad hair day" in one word:. . . . .

I can make a "bad hair day" better by: . . . .

. . . .

Some new strategies I will try when I have a "bad hair day" are:

. . . .

TRUE EMOTIONS COME THROUGH

Purpose of the activity

- To identify and express emotions and feelings in a positive manner
- To develop healthy coping skills and self-regulation
- To identify how emotions impact various aspects of life

Materials needed

- Art canvas, heavy art paper, or water color paper
- Bleeding art tissue paper in assorted colors (this may have to be purchased through a specialist craft store)
- Scissors
- Water
- Large paint brushes

Description of the activity

Begin by asking the participant if he has ever had an emotion that he tried to hide or keep others from seeing. Discuss if he was able to keep the emotion hidden at all times or if the emotion eventually came though. Explain that he is going to create an art project that will provide an example of how "true emotions come through." Provide the participant with all the needed materials. Ask him to select several colors of tissue paper to represent various emotions. Some possibilities might be red for anger, blue for sad, yellow for happy, etc. The participant can choose whatever colors he wants to represent his feelings and emotions. Ask him to cut the tissue paper into a variety of sizes and shapes representing how much time he spends feeling each emotion. For example, if red represents anger and the participant feels angry frequently, then he would cut a large piece of red tissue paper to represent anger. Next, ask him to brush the entire canvas with water using the large paint brush. Once the canvas is wet, have the participant place the strips of tissue paper all over the canvas. If desired, the tissue paper can also be layered on top of other bits of tissue paper in some places to represent times when the participant might experience mixed emotions. After he has arranged all of the tissue paper on the canvas as he chooses, ask him to brush water over the top using the paintbrush. This should be done very lightly so that the tissue paper is not moved from its place on the canvas. Allow the tissue paper to dry completely and then remove it from the canvas. The colors from the tissue paper will have bled through onto the canvas, making a beautiful piece of art.

Variations of the activity

- This activity also works well using different shapes for the canvas, such as hearts and stars.

Discussion questions

- What emotions are represented on your True Emotions Come Through artwork?

- Is one emotion predominant or are there a variety of emotions represented on the artwork?

- Have you ever had an emotion or feeling (such as anger, sadness, etc.) that you tried to hide from others?

- Were you able to keep your emotion successfully hidden from others at all times? How did you do this?

- Sometimes when a person feels angry, they may take out their anger on other people instead of the person they are really angry or upset with. Have you ever done this or observed someone else do this?

- What are some reasons that we might take our anger and frustration out on others (even if they are not the people we are really angry with)?

- Have you ever experienced mixed emotions (feeling two emotions at one time, such as being angry and sad)? What was this like?

- Even when we try to keep our emotions hidden from others, they usually show through as we go about our day. What are some reasons that we may not be able to keep our emotions hidden from others?

- What are some positive ways to express feelings and emotions?

- What happens to anger, sadness, and other emotions if we keep them "hidden" or stuck inside us?

- What are some positive and healthy ways to cope with feelings such as anger and sadness?

- What happened to the tissue paper feelings and emotions when water was added to them? (They bled through onto the canvas.) How does this represent how our feelings and emotions bleed through or come through in our lives?

- What does the completed True Emotions Come Through artwork look like? (It is a beautiful piece of art.) How does this represent expressing our feelings and emotions in life in a healthy and positive manner? (When expressed in a healthy and positive manner, feelings are a beautiful part of life.)

- What is one new coping skill that you can try to cope with your emotions?

- What did you like about creating this artwork?

- What was challenging about creating this artwork?

- What did you learn from completing this artwork?

WE ALL BLEND TOGETHER COLOR WHEEL

Purpose of the activity

- To appreciate individual differences
- To promote positive social skills and communication skills
- To develop group unity

Materials needed

- Large art canvas
- Paint brushes
- Bleeding art tissue paper (one color per participant)
- Water
- Scissors
- Spray bottle
- Pencil
- Ruler or yardstick

Description of the activity

Before the participants arrive, trace a large circle very lightly on the canvas using the pencil. Using the yardstick or ruler, lightly draw lines to make sections on the circle. The number of sections on the circular color wheel should equal the number of participants in the group. When the participants arrive, explain that they are going to work together to create a color wheel. Allow each group member to select a color of tissue paper to use as the project is created. Colors of tissue paper could also be assigned to each group member if that works better for the group. Ask the participants to tear or cut their tissue paper into pieces or shapes. Using the paint brushes and water, completely brush the color wheel circle with water. Next, assign each participant a section on the color wheel. Ask the participant to place and layer his pieces of tissue paper in the assigned section of the color wheel. When all the participants have completed this step, they can carefully (so the tissue paper is not moved) brush back over their section with water or they can use the spray bottle to spray the color wheel with water. Allow the tissue paper to dry completely before removing it.

Variations of the activity

- The completed project makes a beautiful display. If desired, it can be given the heading "We All Blend Together."
- This project can also be completed using other materials. Instead of bleeding tissue paper and water, participants can use colored paper and glue. Paint could also be used.

Discussion questions

- What was it like working so closely with the other group members?

- Were there any challenges with working so closely together on the We All Blend Together Color Wheel? If so, how did you work these challenges out in order to complete the project?

- How did you communicate with the other members of the group to complete the We All Blend Together Color Wheel?

- How does the color wheel represent each group member individually as well as the group as a whole?

- Describe the final result of the We All Blend Together Color Wheel.

- When the tissue paper is removed from the color wheel, do the colors blend together at the intersection of each color? How does this represent the way the group interacts?

- What would the color wheel look like if there was only one color?

- How long would it have taken only one person to create the color wheel without the help of the other group members?

- What are some positive ways that the group can "blend" together and work as a team?

- What is something positive that each person contributes to the group?

- What is something that you learned about yourself or the group as a result of working together to create the We All Blend Together Color Wheel?

BUTTERFLIES IN MY STOMACH

Purpose of the activity

- To identify and understand feelings of anxiety, worry, and nervousness
- To learn positive coping skills
- To encourage positive self-expression and communication skills

Materials needed

- Paper plates
- Large craft or popsicle sticks
- Paint or markers
- Paint brushes (if using paint)
- Buttons or pom poms
- Tacky glue
- Scissors
- Pipe cleaners

Description of the activity

Begin by asking the participant if he has ever heard the expression "I have butterflies in my stomach." This expression is typically used to describe someone who feels nervous, anxious, or maybe even worried about something. Ask the individual to describe some scenarios that make him feel nervous or worried. Discuss some positive ways to cope with worry and anxiety. Provide the participant with the needed supplies. Ask the individual to cut the paper plate into four equal sections. Allow him to paint or color these four sections as desired. These sections will be the butterfly wings. On the back side of each section, ask the participant to write one positive way to cope with worry, anxiety, or feeling nervous. He can also paint the craft stick (which will be the center of the butterfly) or glue buttons or pom poms down the craft stick. The pipe cleaners can be cut into small pieces to serve as the butterfly's antennae. To assemble the butterfly, glue two of the paper plate sections to each side of the craft stick. Next, glue the pipe cleaner antennae to the back of the craft stick. Discuss the coping skills that the participant listed on each butterfly wing.

Variations of the activity

- This is also a good activity for groups.
- Instead of using this activity to discuss anxiety and worry, a "social butterfly" could be created to discuss social skills using the same instructions as above.
- For a fun snack idea to go along with this activity, put some grapes or crackers in a small Ziploc plastic bag. Clip in the middle of the bag with a brightly colored clothespin so

that the two sides of the plastic bag resemble a butterfly's wings and the clothespin serves as the body of the butterfly. Glue pipe cleaners on top of the clothespin (if desired) to serve as the butterfly's antennae. Tell the participant that there is a special snack today to take care of the "butterflies in his stomach."

Discussion questions

- What does the expression "I have butterflies in my stomach" mean?

- Have you ever felt like you had "butterflies in your stomach?" Describe how you felt.

- What does it mean to feel anxious or worried? Describe a time when you felt anxious or worried.

- What does it mean to feel nervous? Tell me about a time when you felt nervous.

- What can you do to handle anxiety or worry in a positive manner?

- How do you cope when you feel nervous about a situation or event?

- Tell me about some of the positive coping skills that you listed on the back of your butterfly wings.

- How can you practice using your positive coping skills when you feel anxious, nervous, or worried?

- What is one new coping skill that you learned today that you can try when you feel anxious, worried, or nervous?

- What is one thing you learned from this activity?

CONNECTING THE DOTS

Purpose of the activity

- To understand the importance of friendships and other relationships

- To encourage positive social skills

- To promote creativity, self-expression, and communication skills

Materials needed

- Paint

- Paint brushes

- Art paper or canvas

Description of the activity

Begin by providing the participant with the needed materials. Ask the individual to put dots of paint around his art paper. The dots should not touch each other. Ask the individual what he notices about the dots of paint. One thing to point out would be that the dots are separated from each other. Each dot is alone. Another thing to discuss would be if the paint is reaching its full potential when it is just a dot. The paint can become a work of art instead of just being a dot. Ask the participant to imagine that he is one of the dots. Ask him to imagine that the other dots are people who he knows, such as family, friends, and others. Discuss some of the things that might keep us as humans separated from each other, such conflict, physical distance, fear, and distrust. Discuss the impact of loneliness and isolation. Next, ask the participant to expand the dots of paint on the art paper or canvas so that the paint begins to spread out and the colors touch each other. Allow the individual to continue this process until all the paint is spread is out and the art paper or canvas is completely covered. Discuss with the individual what is different about the paint now. Point out that all of the dots are spread out and connected. Discuss whether the paint is more beautiful now that it has been spread out, connected with the other colors, and serving a purpose instead of just being an isolated dot. Explain that people also tend to be more beautiful and healthy when they are connected to one other and serving others. The individual can take the painting home as a reminder to value friendships and other people.

Variations of the activity

- This activity works well in groups.

- This activity is great for teens.

- As a variation for groups, the group could complete the activity together instead of individually. Using one large piece of paper, each group member could have one paint color and make a dot to represent himself. After the group discussion, each individual could spread his dot of paint out so that all the colors are connected. This painting makes a beautiful display for the group meeting area.

Discussion questions

After putting dots of paint on the paper:

- What do you notice about the dots of paint?

- Are the dots of paint connected to each other?

- Is the paint serving its highest purpose when it is just a dot on the paper? What else could the paint do?

- Imagine that the dots are people. Are they connected in any way?

- Do we need friendships and relationships with others? Why or why not?

- What are some problems that may happen if we isolate ourselves from others?

- Why is it important to be connected with other people?

- Has social media made us more or less connected with others? Explain your answer.

- What are some ways to choose friends who will be a positive and uplifting influence?

- How can you handle conflicts or problems in friendships and relationships without ending the relationship?

After completing the painting:

- Is the paint more beautiful and purposeful now that it has spread out and is touching the other paint colors? Explain your answer.

- How does the painting represent friendships and relationships with others?

- What are some positive ways to stay connected with other people?

- How can we show others that we value them and the friendships that we have with them?

- Where can you display your Connecting the Dots painting to remind you to stay connected with others and value your positive friendships?

- What is something new that you learned through completing the Connecting the Dots painting that you can apply to your friendships and relationships?

REMINDER RINGS

Purpose of the activity

- To develop positive thinking skills and anger management skills
- To create a visual reminder of therapeutic concepts that will be easily accessible to the individual
- To improve self-concept and self-esteem

Materials needed

- Copies of the Positive Affirmations Reminder Ring Handout and the Anger Management Reminder Ring Handout (these could be printed on heavy-weight paper for durability or colored paper if desired)
- Scissors
- Hole puncher
- Markers, crayons, colored pencils
- Key ring, ring clasp, yarn, or ribbon
- Access to a laminating machine

Description of the activity

Ahead of time, choose whether the participant will make a Reminder Ring for positive affirmations or anger management, or both. This choice can be made based on the needs of the participant or the focus of the sessions. Based on which Reminder Ring the participant will create, the discussion at the beginning of the session should focus on the importance of positive thinking or utilizing anger management strategies. Explain to the participant that it can be easy to list strategies and discuss what to do in certain situations while in the session, but sometimes it can be hard to stay focused on positive thoughts or remember what to do when he is feeling angry outside the session. Provide the participant with the appropriate handout and other needed materials. Assist him in identifying and adding a few personal strategies to either the Positive Affirmations Handout or the Anger Management Handout based on which Reminder Ring he is creating. Allow the participant to color, write on, or decorate the handout. Next, laminate the handout if possible. If you do not have access to a laminator, just continue on to the next step. Once laminated, cut along each of the lines to create eight rectangles. Punch holes in the top left corner of each rectangle. Connect all of the rectangles together using one of the following: a key ring, a ring clasp, yarn or ribbon. Discuss with the participant ways to use his Reminder Ring outside the session to help him remember to utilize his positive thinking skills and anger management skills.

Variations of the activity

- The participant can keep the Reminder Ring in his pocket, desk, or clipped inside a binder. Girls could put their Remind Rings in their purse for easy access.

- Reminder Rings can be created for almost any topic, including social skills, conflict resolution, following directions, rules and expectations.

- This activity also works well with groups. The group could create a Reminder Ring for a topic that has been discussed during group sessions. Together, the participants could create strategies to list on each of the rectangles of the Reminder Ring. This way, the group members gain insight and feedback from each other and learn new strategies to address the issue.

Discussion questions for the Positive Affirmations Reminder Ring Handout

- What does it mean to think positively?

- What is a positive affirmation?

- What are some of the negative thoughts that you struggle with?

- What are some positive affirmations that you could use to replace the negative thoughts?

- When you are outside our sessions do you ever struggle with remembering or utilizing some of the strategies and skills that we discuss? If so, how do you handle this issue?

- What are some ways that you can use your Positive Affirmations Reminder Ring to help you remember to think positively?

- Where will you keep your Positive Affirmations Reminder Ring so that it is easily accessible for you to use?

Discussion questions for the Anger Management Reminder Ring Handout

- What are some of the signs that you are feeling angry?

- How do you cope when you feel angry?

- What are some of the strategies that you use to manage your anger and prevent it from escalating?

- Outside our sessions do you ever have difficulty remembering your anger management strategies and the things we have discussed? If so, what happens when you cannot remember your strategies?

- What are some ways that you can use your Anger Management Reminder Ring to assist you in remembering your strategies when you feel angry or upset?

- Where will you keep your Anger Management Reminder Ring so that it will be easily accessible for you to use?

Positive Affirmations
Reminder Ring Handout

Fill in personal positive affirmations in the blank rectangles, cut out the rectangles, punch a hole in the top left corner, and connect together with a ring clasp or yarn.

My Positive Affirmations Reminder Ring	I love myself
I have lots of positive qualities	I am thankful for all the good things in my life
I am kind to others	I will try my best each day

Anger Management Reminder Ring Handout

Fill in personal anger management strategies in the blank rectangles, cut out the rectangles, punch a hole in the top left corner, and connect together with a ring clasp or yarn.

My Anger Management Reminder Ring	Stop and take a deep breath
Count to ten before speaking	Ask for a break
Walk away	Tell an adult

RACE CAR ART

Purpose of the activity

- To discuss and learn ways to exhibit positive self-control
- To identify the impact of poor self-control and not following directions
- To promote communication skills and social skills

Materials needed

- Large piece of paper or poster-board
- Paint
- Black marker
- Masking tape
- Small Matchbox race cars
- Wipes or water to clean the car wheels
- Newspaper or covering to protect the table or floor

Description of the activity

In advance of the session, use the black marker to draw two race tracks horizontally across the paper or poster-board. The tracks should include a lane wide enough for the Matchbox race cars to fit in. Tape the paper or poster-board to the table or floor (covered to protect the surface from paint stains) where the activity will be completed so that the paper does not move when the cars are raced. When the participant arrives, explain that today he will be using the race cars to learn about impulse control and following directions. Ask him to select a race car. Begin by asking him to race the car down one of the tracks while holding on to the car the entire time. Discuss the following questions with the participant:

- Did you follow directions and hold the car while racing it down the track? If not, what happened?
- Did the car stay on the track while you were holding it?
- Were you in control of the car the entire time?

Next, ask the participant to line the car up on the race track and have the surface tilted slightly to aid the motion of the car so that it will go further. (In this case it would be better done on a table rather than the floor.) Then send it racing on its own down the race tracks instead of holding it the entire time. The participant will have to give it a good shove. Discuss the following questions with the participant:

- Was anything different between this race and the first race when you held the car the entire time? What was it?
- Did the car stay on the race track the entire race? If not, why do you think it went off the track?

- How could these two races compare to our behavior?

- What does our behavior look like when we follow directions and maintain self-control?

- What does our behavior look like when we just take off, racing out of control?

Allow the participant to repeat the races, but this time, ask him to dip the wheels of the car in the paint before completing each race. Discuss the following after both races (one holding on to the car and one with the car racing off on its own):

- What do you notice about the paint tracks left by the car from each race?

- Based on the paint, which car completed the race by staying on the race track the entire time? Which car didn't stay on the race track? How do you explain this?

- Which method of racing works better (to go slower but stay in control or to take off racing fast but then lose control)? Does it work the same way with our behavior?

Allow the participant to race a few more times while continuing to discuss the importance of exhibiting self-control with behavior and being able to follow directions.

Variations of the activity

- This activity also works well with groups. If the activity is being completed with a group, each group member will need his or her own paper and race car.

- Individuals can also be given a blank sheet of paper and several colors of paint. Put the paper on top of newspaper or another covering to protect the floor or table. Ask the individual to dip the wheels of the car in paint and race it across the paper. This can be repeated with the different colors of paint going across the page for a fun activity.

- Another variation includes giving the participant two pieces of paper and a variety of paint colors. On one of the pieces of paper, ask the participant to dip the race car into the paint and let it race across the paper without holding on to it. Ask him to repeat this process with the different colors of paint and starting the car at different corners and locations on the paper. Next, ask him to dip the car in paint and race it across the second piece of paper while holding on to the car the entire time. Ask him to repeat the process using the different paint colors and starting the car at the different locations on the paper, but continuing to hold the car the entire time. When finished, compare both the papers. What are the differences between the patterns of paint on the two pieces of paper? Why do you think the two projects look so different? What can we learn about self-control and behavior from these two art projects? These make great displays for bulletin boards with the heading "Race Car Art."

Discussion questions

- What is self-control?

- What is impulse control?

- Why is it important to follow directions?

- What are some of the differences between the race car that was in control the entire race and the race car that raced out of control?

- Which car stayed on the track and won the race? Why?

- Which method of racing worked the best? Why?

- Were you surprised that the faster car did not win the race? How does this relate to our behavior?

- What are some ways to exhibit more self-control with your behavior?

- What are some ways to do a better job at following directions?

- What are some lessons or observations we can make about self-control and behavior based on this activity?

- What is one new strategy that you can try to improve your self-control in relation to your behavior?

- What is one new strategy that you can try to improve your ability to follow directions?

- What did you like about this activity?

- What did you learn from this activity?

CHAPTER 4

Month-by-Month Character Education Activities

January
PUTTING MY BEST FOOT FORWARD IN THE NEW YEAR

Purpose of the activity

- To identify goals for the new year
- To develop goal-setting and decision-making skills
- To promote positive thinking and creativity

Materials needed

- Paper
- Copies of the Goal-Setting Handout
- Pencils
- Markers
- Materials for collage (old magazines and other sources of images)
- Scissors
- Glue

Description of the activity

Begin by asking the group if they have ever heard the expression "Putting my best foot forward." Explain that this phrase means to do your best, try hard, and work to make a good impression. Discuss with the participants some ways that they can "put their best foot forward in the new year." Assist each of the participants in identifying goals and listing them in the appropriate area on the Goal-Setting Handout. Once the participants have developed their goals, provide them with the other supplies for the activity. Ask each individual to trace his or her foot on the paper. This could be done with or without their socks and shoes on, based on the setting and preferences of the group members. After the participants have finished tracing their feet, ask them to use the collage materials to find images to represent the goals that they listed on their Goal-Setting Handout. The participants will cut these images out and glue them inside the outlines of their feet. They can also use the markers to draw or write words to represent their goals. When complete, the foot outline can be cut out using the scissors. Allow each participant to tell the group about his or her "foot" and the ways that he or she will "put their best foot forward in the new year."

Variations of the activity

- This is also a great activity to use at the beginning of the school year.

- These make a nice bulletin board or group display with the heading "Putting My Best Foot Forward in the New Year."

- Participants can keep their Goal-Setting Handouts in a binder or similar place so that they can frequently refer to them and stay focused on achieving their goals. They can also display their foot collage in a frequently viewed spot as a visual reminder of their goals for the year.

Discussion questions

- What does the expression "Putting my best foot forward" mean?

- Why is it important to start the new year off on your "best foot?"

- How is the new year an opportunity to start fresh and make positive changes?

- What are some of your goals for this year in different areas of your life?

- Why should we set goals for ourselves?

- What are some steps that you will need to take this year to achieve the goals that you have identified?

- What is one thing that you will need to do differently this year in order to achieve the goals that you have set for yourself?

- Tell me about the images, words, or drawings that you included on your best foot forward artwork.

- What did you like about this activity?

- What was challenging about this activity?

- What did you learn from participating in this activity?

Goal-Setting Handout

Goal for physical health:. . . . .

. . . .

Goal for mental health:. . . . .

. . . .

Goal for behavior:. . . . .

. . . .

Goal for relationships:. . . . .

. . . .

Goal for education:. . . . .

. . . .

Goal for recreation:. . . . .

. . . .

Goal for giving back to others:. . . . .

. . . .

IMPROVING OUR WORLD HANDPRINT WREATH (DR. MARTIN LUTHER KING JR.'S BIRTHDAY)

Purpose of the activity

- To develop positive social skills
- To develop conflict resolution skills
- To promote communication, empathy, and self-awareness

Materials needed

- Brief biography of Dr. Martin Luther King Jr. (www.thekingcenter.org/about-dr-king)
- Construction paper
- Pencils
- Scissors
- Markers
- Glue
- Large piece of paper or poster-board
- Masking tape

Description of the activity

Begin by giving the participants some information about Dr. Martin Luther King Jr. (born January 15, 1929) and his accomplishments. In particular, discuss ways that he tried to make the world a better place. In addition, discuss ways that Dr. King tried to promote peaceful conflict resolution, positive social interactions, empathy, respect for others, and communication. Explain that we can all continue Dr. King's legacy by trying to make our world a better place each day and influencing the people around us in a positive way. Ask participants to spend a few minutes thinking about how they can make a difference in their world (classroom, home, relationships with others) in the following areas:

- Peaceful conflict resolution
- Positive social interactions
- Empathy for others
- Respect for others
- Communication.

Distribute the supplies to the participants. Ask each participant to trace their hand on the construction paper and then use the scissors to cut out the handprint. Next, ask the participants to write their names in the palms of their handprints and write some of the ways that they can have a hand in making the world a better place on the fingers of their handprints. The handprints can be outlined and decorated with the markers. When all the participants have completed their handprints, ask each one to share the ways that they can have a hand in making the world a better place. Tape the large paper or poster-board (with the heading "We All Have a Hand in Making the World a Better Place") to a wall. After each participant shares the information from their handprint, ask them to come and attach it to the poster-board. The handprints should be placed side by side (fingers facing out) to form the shape of a wreath or circle. Discuss some of the common ideas, concepts, and behaviors that participants listed on their handprints and the practical ways that the participants can exhibit these behaviors on a daily basis.

Variations of the activity

- This makes a great display for the group area or classroom. The handprint wreath can serve as a daily visual reminder for the participants that they have a hand in making their world a better place.

- The handprint wreath and "We All Have a Hand in…" theme can be applied to many different topics and holidays. For example, "We All Have a Hand in Following the Rules" or "We All Have a Hand in Showing Love for Others (Valentine's Day)."

Discussion questions

- Tell me about Dr. Martin Luther King Jr. and some of the reasons that we celebrate his legacy each year on his birthday.

- What were some of the ways that Dr. King promoted peaceful conflict resolution?

- What were some of the ways that he promoted positive social interactions among all people?

- What were some of the ways that Dr. King promoted empathy and respect for others?

- What were some of the ways that Dr. King promoted communication among all people?

- How can you have a "hand" in continuing Dr. King's legacy and making your world a better place?

- What are some ways that you can promote peaceful conflict resolution at home and at school?

- What are some ways that you can promote positive social interactions with the people that you see each day?

- What are some ways that you can show empathy and respect to the people you encounter each day?

- What are some ways that you can promote positive communication with the people you spend time with each day?

- Please tell us about your handprint and the things that you wrote on your handprint.

After completing the handprint wreath:

- What are some things that you notice about the handprint wreath? (All the handprints are connected to each other.)

- What would the handprint wreath look like if there was only one hand on the wreath?

- How can our handprint wreath serve as a reminder to us to display the characteristics we have discussed today and work to make the world around us a better place?

- What did you like about creating the handprint wreath?

- What was challenging about creating the handprint wreath?

- What did you learn from creating the handprint wreath?

February
STRING OF HEARTS (VALENTINE'S DAY)

Purpose of the activity

- To develop positive social skills
- To express kindness to others
- To promote positive thinking and communication skills

Materials needed

- Construction paper
- Yarn or ribbon
- Scissors
- Markers
- Hole puncher

Description of the activity

In advance of the group, use the scissors to cut hearts out of the construction paper. The hearts should be about five inches in length. Each participant will need a set of hearts equal to the number of participants in the group. For example, if there are ten participants, then each participant will need ten hearts. If time allows, the participants could cut out their own heart shapes. Explain to the group that Valentine's Day is a day associated with showing love and kindness to others. Ask the group to identify some different ways to show love and kindness to others. Some of the ways that we show love and kindness might include using positive and uplifting words, giving gifts, doing acts of kindness, and spending time with those we love. Tell the participants that today they are going to show love and kindness to the other members of the group by using kind words. Ask the participants to write the name of each group member on one of their hearts. Ask them to write one positive thing about the group member on the other side of the heart. Each participant can also make a heart for him or herself and write something positive about him or herself on the heart. I always enjoy participating in this activity and making a heart for each group member, listing a positive trait that I have observed about each member. Once all of the participants have completed their hearts, they can punch a hole in the top center of each heart. Next, the participants can distribute the hearts to the other group members. Once each group member has received the hearts with the positive statements, provide each group member with a long piece of string or ribbon. They can then thread the string through the holes in their hearts to create a garland of hearts. The hearts may need to be knotted on the garland so that they hold in place. When all the group members have completed their garland, discuss the activity.

Variations of the activity

- Instead of a garland of hearts, a book of hearts could be created. Instead of a long piece of yarn or ribbon, provide participants with a short piece and tie the hearts together.

- After the activity, the group could have a Celebration of Kindness party for Valentine's Day to practice using positive social skills and manners. Consider serving only red and pink food to go along with the Valentine's Day theme.

Discussion questions

- What are some of the themes often associated with Valentine's Day?

- What are some reasons that we should be kind and show love to others?

- What are some of the different ways that we can show love and kindness to others?

- How do you feel when someone says something kind to you or gives you a compliment?

- How do you feel when you say something kind or do something kind for someone else?

- Why is it important to take the time to say kind things to others?

- What was it like receiving the String of Hearts garland with all of the kind words from the other group members?

- How did you feel as you were reading the kind words and positive statements that others wrote about you?

- How did you feel about writing the positive statements about the other group members on the hearts and then giving them the hearts?

- What is one new way that you can try to show more kindness and love to those around you each day?

- What did you like about creating the String of Hearts garland?

- What did you learn from participating in this activity?

PIECES OF MY HEART MOSAIC (VALENTINE'S DAY)

Purpose of the activity

- To identify and express feelings in a healthy manner
- To identify important relationships in each group member's life
- To identify positive ways to show kindness to others

Materials needed

- Construction paper (assorted colors)
- Large red hearts (cut from construction paper)
- Scissors
- Glue
- Copies of the Pieces of My Heart Handout
- Pencils
- Crayons, markers

Description of the activity

Begin by discussing Valentine's Day and some of the common associations that we make with the day. One of the most common symbols of Valentine's Day is the heart. Ask the individuals to think about some of the things that are in their "hearts" right now. It could be feelings of happiness, anger, sadness, or a mixture of emotions. It could be thoughts concerning relationships with others including family and friends, or other significant relationships. It could be anxiety or worries. It could be excitement about upcoming events. Explain to the group that they are going to make heart mosaics to represent the mixture of emotions, thoughts, and relationships that are in their hearts right now. Provide the group members with the needed supplies. Ask them to select a different color of construction paper to represent each of the different emotions, thoughts, or relationships that are in their hearts now. For example, pink might represent love, blue might represent sadness, yellow might represent friendships, black might represent worry or grief, etc. The participants can choose the meanings for each color as desired and then list what each color means on their Pieces of My Heart Handout. After completing this step, the group members can cut the colored construction paper into pieces and then glue these onto the heart to represent the amount of space that each thought or feeling takes up in their hearts. For example, if one of the participants feels happy a lot (represented by pink) and values his or her friendships (represented by yellow), then he or she would have lots of pink and yellow pieces glued to his or her heart. The entire heart should be covered with pieces of construction paper when complete. Once all of the group members have completed their hearts, discuss what each heart represents and ways to show kindness to those who are in our hearts and around us.

Variations of the activity

- This activity also works well for individual sessions.
- The completed mosaics make a great display for bulletin boards or group spaces with the heading "These are the Pieces of Our Hearts."
- For a fun snack, serve Reese's Pieces on heart-shaped plates after completing the activity.

Discussion questions

- How is the heart associated with Valentine's Day?
- What does the heart represent?
- What are some of the feelings, emotions, thoughts, and relationships that are in your heart right now?
- How did you choose which colors would represent which feelings, thoughts, or relationships?
- Tell me about your Pieces of My Heart Mosaic.
- What could we learn about you by looking at your Pieces of My Heart Mosaic?
- How do you feel about your completed Pieces of My Heart Mosaic?
- Is there anything you want change or anything that you are struggling with in your heart right now? Explain your answer.
- What are some ways that you can show kindness and love to the people in the relationships with you that are represented on your heart?
- How can we let others know that we value them?
- What did you like about completing this activity?
- What was challenging about completing this activity?
- What did you learn from completing this activity?

Pieces of My Heart Handout

In the blank next to each color, list the feeling, thought, relationship, or other aspect it will represent on your Pieces of My Heart Mosaic

Red = ...

Blue = ...

Yellow = ...

Pink = ...

White = ...

Black = ...

Orange = ...

Green = ...

Gray = ...

Purple = ...

Brown = ...

Other = ...

March

RAINBOW OF DIFFERENT COLORS (ST. PATRICK'S DAY)

Purpose of the activity

- To develop group unity and cohesiveness
- To appreciate and understand similarities and differences among people
- To develop empathy and tolerance for others

Materials needed

- Copies of the Rainbow of Different Colors Handout (laminated)
- Assorted colors of playdough or modeling clay

Description of the activity

Begin by asking the group members about some common associations and traditions related to St. Patrick's Day. One of the common themes of St. Patrick's Day is the rainbow. Ask the group to tell you about rainbows. Be sure that someone points out that a rainbow has many different colors. Provide the group members with the Rainbow of Different Colors Handouts and playdough or modeling clay. Ask each individual to fill in the lines of the rainbow with a different color of the playdough. Each group member's rainbow should have multiple colors of playdough on it representing all the different colors in the rainbow. Discuss the following questions:

- What does the playdough feel like in your hands?
- Did the different colors of playdough feel different in your hands? Why not?
- What do you notice about your playdough rainbows?
- How many different colors are represented on your rainbow?
- What would it look like if there was only one color on the rainbow? Would it still be a rainbow?

Next, begin to discuss differences among people with the group using the rainbow as a metaphor.

- How does the rainbow represent the differences and similarities among people?
- How does the playdough represent the ways that people are all similar? How does the playdough also represent individual differences between people?
- What makes the rainbow so beautiful? How does this relate to our group?

- What are some of the special traits and qualities that the other members bring to the group that you appreciate?

- How can we celebrate the differences between us instead of criticizing others for being different?

Conclude by asking each group member to share a way that they can encourage and appreciate differences and promote unity in their world.

Variations of the activity

- If playdough or modeling clay is not available, this activity could also be completed as a mosaic using assorted colors of construction paper or tissue paper glued to the handout.

- After completing the activity, consider having a special party to celebrate St. Patrick's Day with rainbow-colored snacks, green punch, or Lucky Charms cereal.

Discussion questions

- What are some common associations and symbols of St. Patrick's Day?

- What is a rainbow?

- What are some of the special features of a rainbow?

- What does the word "different" mean?

- How is our group different? How is our group alike?

- Would the rainbow be as beautiful if there was only one color? How do the different colors in the rainbow make it more beautiful?

- Even though there were several different colors of playdough or modeling clay, they all felt alike and could all be part of the rainbow. What are some ways that all people are alike?

- How can you show respect for others who may be "different" from you?

- How is the rainbow a metaphor or visual example of our group?

- How is the rainbow a metaphor or visual example of the world?

- What is one new way that you can show respect for the differences among the people you are with each day?

- What is one new way that you can promote unity and relationship with the other group members?

- What did you like about completing this activity?

- What was challenging about completing this activity?

- What did you learn from completing this activity?

Rainbow of Different Colors Handout

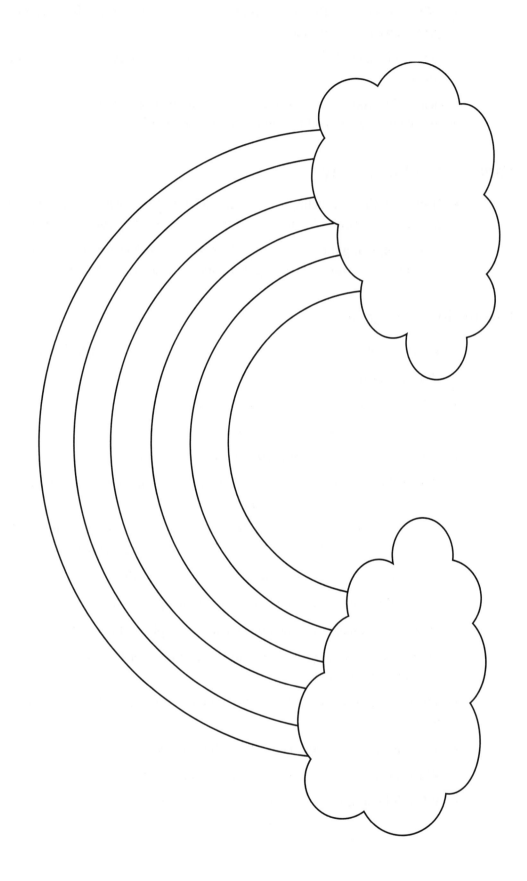

POT OF GOLD GOALS COLLAGE (ST. PATRICK'S DAY)

Purpose of the activity

- To identify goals and steps to take to accomplish goals
- To promote self-awareness, communication skills, and creativity
- To develop positive thinking skills

Materials needed

- Copies of the Pot of Gold Goals Collage Handout
- Collage materials (old magazines and other sources of images)
- Scissors
- Glue
- Markers
- Pencils
- Paper

Description of the activity

Begin by discussing St. Patrick's Day and some of the common symbols and traditions associated with the day. St. Patrick's Day is an Irish holiday celebrated each year on March 17th. One common Irish symbol is the pot of gold found at the end of the rainbow. Some traditions and legends also discuss leprechauns that hide the pots of gold at the end of the rainbow. Ask the group members to think about what their personal pots of gold might look like. Discuss the following with them:

- What would your personal pot of gold look like?
- Would it include getting married and having children?
- Would it include a successful and fulfilling career?
- Where would you live?
- What would your house look like?
- How would you give back to others?
- What else would be included in your pot of gold?

Distribute the needed materials and ask the group members to find images to make a collage, write words or phrases, or draw pictures to represent their personal pot of gold. When all of the group members have completed the collage, discuss the images that each participant selected and how the images represent his or her "personal pot of gold." Assist the participants in identifying specific steps that they will need to take to reach their goals. Discuss the "leprechauns" that might be obstacles in the way of achieving their goals, and how to overcome these obstacles. Consider ending the group by asking the group members to write a Positive Pot of Gold Goal Statement to summarize the goals that are represented on their collages and the steps that they will have to take to achieve their goals.

Variation of the activity

- This activity also works well for individual sessions.
- These collages make a great display for bulletin boards or group meeting spaces with the heading "Our Pots of Gold are Full of Goals."
- When the activity is complete, have a St. Patrick's Day party with green and rainbow-colored food and drinks.

Discussion questions

- What are some symbols and traditions associated with St. Patrick's Day?
- What does the pot of gold represent?
- What would you include in your personal pot of gold?
- What images, phrases, or drawings did you include on your Pot of Gold Goal Collage?
- What do the images, words, and phrases on your Pot of Gold Goal Collage represent?
- What are some actions and steps that you will need to take to reach your pot of gold goals?
- What is one specific step that you can take toward achieving each of the goals that you identified on your Pot of Gold Goal Collage?
- What are some "leprechauns" or obstacles that might cause challenges or difficulty on the way to achieving your goals?
- How can you overcome the "leprechauns" or obstacles that you may face on the way achieving your goals?
- Please share your Positive Pot of Gold Goal Statement with the group.
- What did you like about creating the collage?
- What was challenging about creating the collage?
- What did you learn from creating the collage?

Pot of Gold Goals Collage Handout

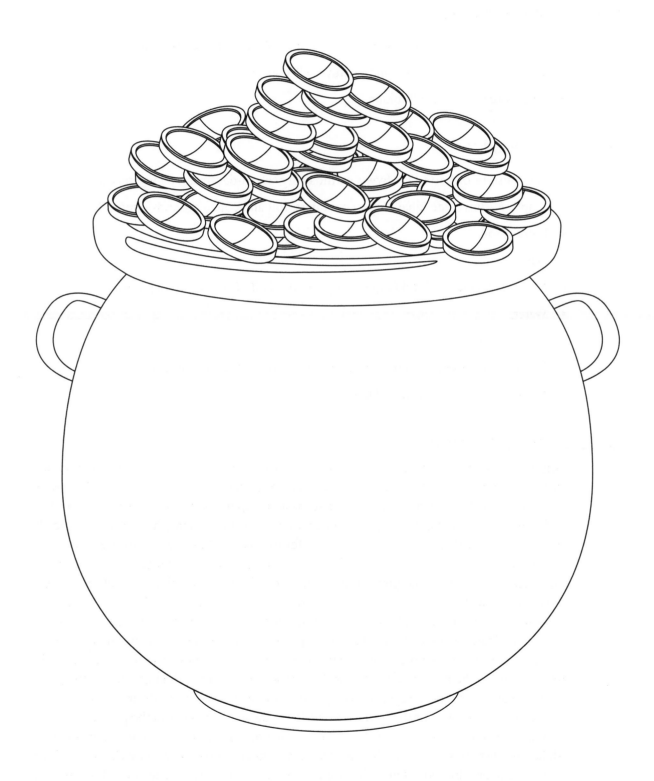

April

GROWING SEEDS OF HEALTH AND WELLNESS (EARTH DAY)

Purpose of the activity

- To identify ways to take care of physical, mental, and emotional health
- To promote self-awareness and positive self-concept
- To encourage positive thinking

Materials needed

- Brief history of Earth Day (www.earthday.org/earth-day-history-movement)
- Empty K-cups (individual coffee containers, foil and coffee grounds removed)
- Potting soil
- Seeds
- Plastic container with lid (large enough to hold all of the K-cup planters)
- Water
- Sharpie markers
- Pencil or other object to poke holes in the bottom of the K-cup planter
- Copies of the Growth Chart Handout

Description of the activity

Begin by asking the group members if they have ever heard of Earth Day and giving them a brief history of Earth Day. Explain that we all have a responsibility to take care of the environment in which we live. We also have a responsibility to take care of ourselves and continue to grow physically, mentally, and emotionally. Discuss how growth typically begins with a small seed and then, as we care for the seed and provide for its needs, the seed grows into food for us to eat, beautiful flowers, trees, plants, etc. Discuss with the group members how our personal growth in the areas of physical, mental, and emotional health often begins with a small step, idea, or "seed" and as we continue to "water" the idea by making positive choices and taking additional steps then we continue to "grow," just like seeds. Distribute the needed materials to the participants. Ask them to write their names on the outside of their K-cup planter using the Sharpie marker. Next, use the pencil to poke several holes in the bottom of the K-cup. Fill the K-cup planter with moistened potting soil. Read the directions for the specific seed packets that you are using to determine how much soil covering is needed for the seeds to grow. Place the K-cup planter in the plastic container with a small amount of water in the bottom, place the lid on top, and put in a warm area. Make sure that the soil stays moist. After the plants begin to sprout, remove the lid but keep them in a sunny location. Once the plants grow to about three inches tall (this will take a couple of weeks), they will need to be transferred to a larger pot. If desired, the group members can report the daily growth of their seed and their personal growth on the Growth Chart Handout.

Variations of the activity

- The seeds could be started in pots, but using the K-cups is a good illustration of how a small step or idea can lead to growth and amazing progress. It is also a good way to discuss how to reuse things that would otherwise be discarded.

- If your group is one that continuously meets, then allowing each group member to care for their plant and watch its growth throughout the group sessions is a great way to teach responsibility.

- This activity could be incorporated as part of a science lesson on plants.

- The growth chart can be completed each day during group time as a means to report the daily progress of the individual's seed as well as any personal growth the individual has observed in his or her life in the areas of physical, mental, or emotional growth. For example, the individual might note that his or her plant has sprouted in the column for "Seed growth" and that he or she used his or her anger control strategies to avoid a fight in the column for "Personal growth." This could serve as a way to begin the group discussion each day.

Discussion questions

- What is Earth Day?

- What are some ways that we can take of the Earth?

- Why is it important for everyone to do their part in caring for the Earth?

- What will we need to plant our seeds?

- What will the seeds need to grow into plants?

- How is our personal growth (physical, mental, and emotional) similar to the growth of a seed into a plant?

- What are some small seeds that you can "plant" in your life in the areas of physical, emotional, and mental growth?

- How can you "water" these physical, mental, and emotional seeds that you have planted so that they will continue to grow?

- What will happen if you do not water your seeds and the seeds dry out?

- What happens in your life when you stop taking care of yourself physically, emotionally, or mentally?

- What are some ways to grow and take care of yourself physically?

- What are some ways to grow and take care of yourself mentally?

- What are some ways to grow and take care of yourself emotionally?

- How often will we need to check on our seeds that we have planted to see if they need water?

- How can you develop responsibility by caring for your seed that you planted?

- Will the seed need a new pot after it grows into a plant? Why?

- Have you ever "outgrown" something in your life as you became more physically, emotionally, or mentally healthy? How did you handle this issue?

- What is one new "seed" (a small idea or step) that you can plant in each area of your life to grow and become more healthy?

- What did you like about planting your seed in your planter?

- What did you learn from participating in this activity and planting your seed?

Growth Chart Handout

Use this chart to document the growth of your seed in the "Seed growth" column and any progress you made in personal growth in the "Personal growth" column.

Date:	Seed growth:	Personal growth:

RELAXATION PLAYDOUGH BALLOONS (SPRING BREAK)

Purpose of the activity

- To build positive coping skills
- To create a sensory object to use when anxious, frustrated, or angry
- To develop anger management skills

Materials needed

- Heavy-weight balloons in assorted colors
- Playdough
- Sharpie markers

Description of the activity

Begin by discussing stress and anxiety with the group. What does it mean to be stressed or anxious? What are some ways to cope with stress and learn to relax? Explain to the group members that they are going to create some Relaxation Balloons that they can use to relax when they feel stressed, anxious or angry. Distribute the needed supplies to the group members. Ask them to fill their balloons with playdough. The easiest way to accomplish this is either to roll the playdough out to the shape of a long cylinder or to break the playdough into small pieces and roll into little balls. Stretch the opening of the balloon as wide as possible and fill with the playdough. It is more efficient to do this in pairs, with one person holding the balloon open and the other person filling the balloon with playdough. Once complete, tie the balloons closed. Next, allow the group members to use the Sharpie markers to write words that will remind them of their anger management strategies. Examples might include "Relax," "Peace," or "Let it Go." The group members may also choose to write their name or create a design on their Relaxation Balloons using the Sharpie markers. Remind them not to press too hard so that they do not tear a hole in the balloon. Discuss ways that they can use their balloons to relax and calm themselves when stressed, anxious, or angry.

Variations of the activity

- The Relaxation Playdough Balloons also work well for individual sessions.
- If you do not have playdough, you could also fill the balloons with rice, salt, or sand.

Discussion questions

- What does it mean to "relax?"
- What is stress?

- How does stress make you feel?

- What are some unhealthy ways that people may cope with stress?

- What are some healthy ways to cope with stress?

- What is anger?

- How do you know when you are angry?

- What are some unhealthy ways to handle anger?

- What are some healthy ways to manage anger?

- What is anxiety?

- What are some unhealthy ways to manage anxiety?

- What are some healthy ways to manage anxiety?

- Why is it important to relax when we are stressed or angry?

- How would someone be able to tell if you were calm and relaxed?

- Describe how it feels to be calm and relaxed.

- What are coping skills? Give some examples of some healthy coping skills.

- How can you use your Relaxation Playdough Balloon to help you cope when you feel stressed, angry, or anxious?

- Where will you keep your Relaxation Playdough Balloon so that you can get to it quickly and easily if you begin to feel stressed, angry, or anxious?

- What did you like about this activity?

- What did you learn from this activity?

May

MOTHER'S DAY FLOWER

Purpose of the activity

- To express gratitude for mothers or maternal figures
- To promote positive thinking and communication skills
- To develop kindness and compassion

Materials needed

- Copies of the Mother's Day Flower Handout
- Small pictures of each participant (to fit inside the circle at the center of each flower)
- Markers, crayons
- Pens
- Scissors
- Glue
- Assorted colors of construction paper
- Access to a laminating machine or sheet protectors

Description of the activity

Begin by asking the group members to think of some of the traits and things that they appreciate about their mother (or a maternal figure for group members who may not have a mother in their life). Explain that Mother's Day is a day to take the time to show appreciation and love to our mothers or the maternal figures in our lives. Provide the group members with the needed supplies. Ask each group member to write one thing he or she loves or appreciates about his or her mother on each of the petals on the Mother's Day Flower Handout. After the group members complete this part, assist them in cutting their pictures into a circular shape that will fit into the center of the flower template. Allow the group members to glue the pictures on to the center of the flower. Next, let each group member lightly (so that the words on each petal are still visible) color and decorate the flower template using his or her mother's favorite colors. When this is complete, assist the group members in cutting out their flower templates and the Mother's Day poem on the Mother's Day Flower Handout and glue the flower and the poem to a piece of construction paper. The group members can write "A Flower for My Mother" at the top of the construction paper. At the bottom of the paper, they can write their name and the year. If possible, laminate the construction paper in order to create a lasting gift when the group members give it to their mothers. If a laminating machine is not available, the construction paper could be placed inside a sheet protector for preservation. Finish by discussing other ways to show love and appreciation to the mothers and maternal figures in their lives throughout the year.

Variations of the activity

- This also works well as an individual activity.

- If you have siblings in the group or more time to complete the activity, a Mother's Day Bouquet of Flowers can be created. Each sibling can create a flower (using the instructions above) and then the flowers can be glued to a large piece of paper and stems can be drawn on to this. If you have more time to complete the activity, each group member can make two or three flowers (using the instructions above) for their mother and create a "bouquet of flowers" for her on a large piece of paper. They can then write "A Bouquet of Flowers for My Mother" at the top of the paper and their name and the year at the bottom of the paper. The Mother's Day poem on the Mother's Day Flower Handout can also be copied on to the large piece of paper if desired.

Discussion questions

- What is Mother's Day?

- Why do we need Mother's Day?

- What are some reasons that we should let our mothers or the maternal figures in our lives know how much we love and appreciate them?

- What are some of the traits and things about your mother (or maternal figure) that you love and appreciate?

- What are some ways that you can show gratitude and love to your mother?

- What are some ways that your mother (or maternal figure) lets you know that she loves you?

- While it is important to show our mothers (or maternal figures) love and appreciation on Mother's Day, it is also important to express our gratitude and love throughout the year. What are some ways that you can show your gratitude and love for your mother throughout the year?

- What is something that you can do to help your mother each day?

- What did you like about completing this activity?

- What did you learn from creating this activity?

Mother's Day Flower Handout

On this Mother's Day,
I have made you a flower listing each way
That I love you so much and appreciate all that you do
This flower will last forever and my love for you will, too.

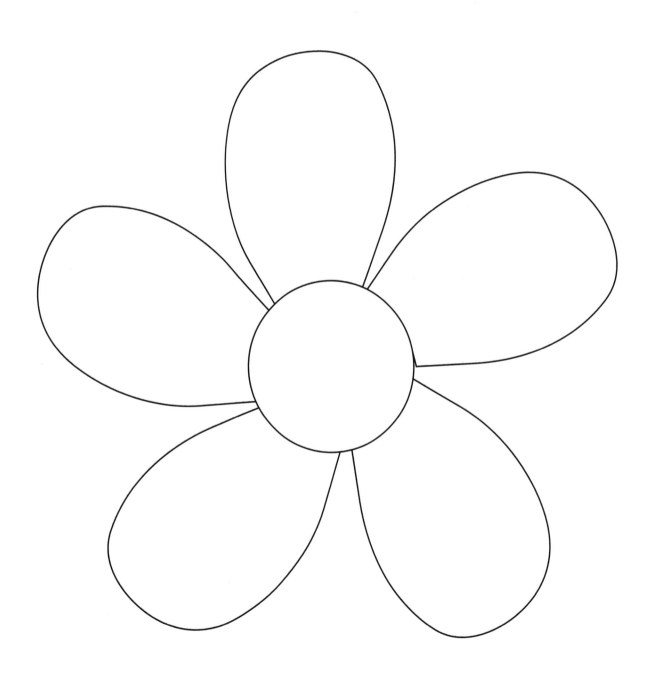

A MOTHER'S DAY INTERVIEW (MOTHER'S DAY)

Purpose of the activity

- To express love and gratitude for mothers or maternal figures

- To encourage positive thinking

- To develop positive listening and communication skills

Materials needed

- Copies of the Mother's Day Interview Handout

- Pens

- Assorted colors of construction paper

- Scissors

- Glue

- Access to a laminating machine or sheet protectors

Description of the activity

Begin by talking with the group about Mother's Day. Ask them to think of some things that they appreciate about their mother (or a maternal figure in their life). Be mindful of group members who may not have a mother in their life and adapt the activity accordingly. Explain to the group that you will be interviewing each of them about their mother. This will provide them with an opportunity to practice their listening skills and communication skills. As you interview the group members, write their responses on the Mother's Day Interview Handout. When complete, ask each group member to select a piece of construction paper. Next, they can cut out the interview and glue it to the construction paper. If possible, laminate the construction paper so that it will be more durable. If you do not have access to a laminating machine, the construction paper can be placed inside a sheet protector to preserve it. The group members can give the completed interviews to their mother as a gift for Mother's Day.

Variations of the activity

- This also works well as an activity for an individual session.

- If the group is short on time, you can have the group members interview each other instead of each group member being interviewed by the group leader. This will save time and allow the group members to practice listening and communication skills with their peers.

- A similar interview could be developed for Father's Day and Grandparents' Day to give as a gift on these special days.

Discussion questions

- What is Mother's Day?

- How can you show your mother (or a maternal figure in your life) that you love and appreciate her?

- Why is it important to let our mothers (and other important people in our life) know that we love and appreciate them?

- What are some ways that you can help your mother each day?

- What did you think about completing the Mother's Day Interview?

- What do you think your mother will think about the Mother's Day Interview that you completed?

- What skills did you have an opportunity to practice while completing the Mother's Day Interview?

- If you completed the interview with a peer, was it easier to ask your partner the questions or answer the questions when your partner interviewed you? Explain your answer.

- What did you like about completing the interview?

- What was challenging about completing the interview?

- What did you learn from completing this activity?

Mother's Day Interview Handout

I love my mother because:. . . . .

My mother is the best because:. . . . .

I am thankful for my mother because:. . . . .

My mother and I are alike because: . . . .

I hope my mother knows: . . . .

I know my mother loves me because: . . . .

I love it when my mother: . . . .

My favorite thing to do with my mother is: . . . .

My mother loves to: . . . .

My mother always knows: . . . .

I am going to help my mother by: . . . .

One thing I want to tell my mother is: . . . .

Interview answers provided by: . . . . ,

Age: . . . . Date: . . . .

June

COOLING DOWN MY ANGER ICE CREAM PARTY (SUMMER)

Purpose of the activity

- To learn to express anger in positive and healthy ways
- To develop anger management skills
- To promote positive coping skills

Materials needed

- Copies of the Cooling Down My Anger Handout
- Markers, pens
- Scissors
- Glue
- Construction paper
- Ice cream
- Ice cream cones

Description of the activity

Begin by discussing summer with the group. Summer is often associated with hot weather or heat. Anger can be associated with feeling hot as well. Explain to the group members that they are going to discuss some ways to "cool down" their anger when they begin to feel hot. Ask the group members to identify some of the signs that they may be feeling angry. Some examples might include red face, clenched fists, gritted teeth, feeling hot, or heavy breathing. Assist the group members in identifying some different ways to "cool down" or prevent their anger from escalating. Some examples might include walking away, asking for a break, deep breathing, counting to ten, or squeezing a stress ball. Distribute the needed materials (except for the ice cream and ice cream cones) to the group members. Ask each group member to write to three anger management strategies that he or she can use on the three swirls of ice cream on the Cooling Down My Anger Handout. Next, ask the group members to color and decorate the ice cream cone on the handout. After completing this step, they will cut out their ice cream cones and glue them to one of the pieces of construction paper. Allow the group members to share the strategies that they listed on their Cooling Down My Anger Handouts and ways that they will use these strategies when they are feeling angry. After all of the group members have shared their strategies, serve the ice cream in cones and have a Cooling Down My Anger Ice Cream Party.

Variations of the activity

- The Cooling Down My Anger ice cream cones on the construction paper make a great display for bulletin boards or group areas with the heading "We're Cooling Down Our Anger This Summer!"

- This activity works well for end of the year parties or Positive Behavioral Interventions and Support (PBIS) reward celebrations.

Discussion questions

- What is the weather like during the summer?

- What are some of the signs or physical symptoms of anger?

- How is heat or feeling hot often associated with anger?

- How do you handle it when you feel angry?

- What are some positive ways to "cool down" your anger and prevent it from escalating?

- What strategies have you tried to manage your anger in the past? Did these strategies work for you? Explain your answer.

- What are some triggers or situations that may make you feel angry?

- How can you use anger management strategies to cope with these triggers or situations in a positive way?

- What anger management strategies did you list on your Cooling Down My Anger Handout?

- How will you use the anger management strategies listed on your Cooling Down My Anger Handout when you feel angry?

- What did you like about this activity?

- What was challenging about this activity?

- What did you learn from participating in this activity?

Cooling Down My Anger Handout

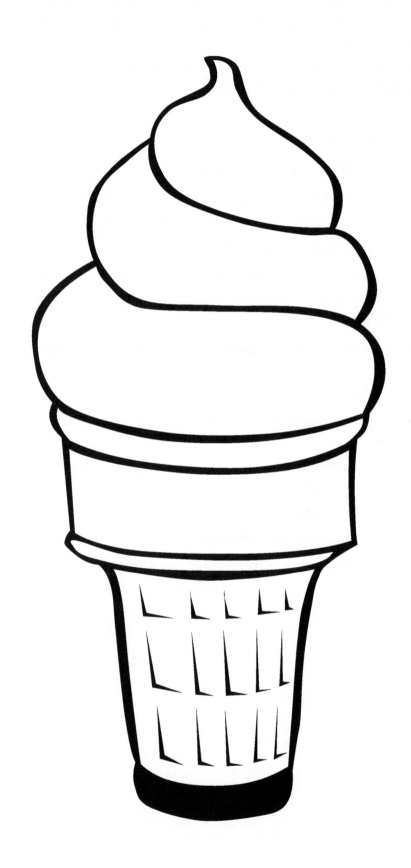

POSITIVE THINKING SUNSHINE (SUMMER)

Purpose of the activity

- To promote positive thinking
- To develop self-awareness and improve self-concept
- To encourage coping skills and communication skills

Materials needed

- Copies of the Positive Thinking Sunshine Handout
- Markers
- Pens, pencils
- Construction paper (yellow)
- Scissors
- Hole puncher
- Yarn, ribbon

Description of the activity

Sunny days are often associated with happiness, optimism, and positive things. Discuss the importance of positive thinking with the group. Ask group members to identify some negative thoughts that they may struggle with in their minds. Ask them to turn the negative thoughts into positive statements or affirmations. Provide assistance to those who may have difficulty in developing positive thoughts or affirmations. Distribute the needed materials to the group members. Ask them to cut out the sunshine template from the Positive Thinking Sunshine Handout and then trace it on to the yellow construction paper and cut it out. Next, ask the group members to write their positive statements or affirmations on the yellow sunshine shape. If desired, the group members can decorate their sunshine shape using the markers. When complete, punch a hole in the top of the sunshine shapes and tie yarn or ribbon through the hole so that the group members can hang them in a place for frequent viewing. Once all the group members have completed the activity, ask them to share the positive statements and affirmations that they wrote on their sunshine shapes and ways that each group member will use the positive statements and affirmations to promote positive thinking.

Variations of the activity

- This is also a good activity for individual sessions.
- The Positive Thinking Sunshine shapes make a great display for bulletin boards or group areas with the title "The Sun is Shining Brightly with Positive Thinking."
- If you are short on time for the activity, the Positive Thinking Sunshine Handout can just be copied onto yellow paper instead of cutting out the template and tracing it onto construction paper.

- This activity can also be completed as a collaborative group project. On a large piece of paper, ask the group members to work together to paint or color with markers a large sunshine shape and its rays on the paper. While the sunshine shape is drying, discuss positive thinking with the group using the discussion questions below. Once the sunshine shape has dried (or in the next group session), give each of the group members pens or markers and ask them to write their positive statements and affirmations around the sunshine shape. When complete, write "Positive Thinking Sunshine" across the top of the paper. This makes a beautiful display. If displayed in the group meeting area, the group leader can ask group members to read a positive statement or affirmation at the beginning or end of each group session to continue to promote positive thinking.

- If you have more time to complete the activity, each group member could paint a sunshine shape on a large piece paper. Once it is dry, the group members can write their positive statements and affirmations around and on their sunshine shapes. They can take their artwork with them to display in a prominent place so that they can view and frequently use their positive statements and affirmations. This variation makes a beautiful project when complete.

Discussion questions

- What are some associations that people make with sunshine?
- How could positive thinking and optimism be associated with sunshine?
- What does it mean to think positively?
- What does it mean to be optimistic?
- What are some negative thoughts or worries that you struggle with inside your head?
- What are some positive statements or affirmations that you can use to replace each negative thought or worry?
- Why is it important to think positively and use positive affirmations?
- What are some of the positive statements and affirmations that you listed on your Positive Thinking Sunshine?
- Where will you hang your Positive Thinking Sunshine so that you can see it often?
- Why is it important to speak our positive thoughts and affirmations aloud?
- How will you use your Positive Thinking Sunshine to remind you to think positively?
- What are some ways that you can use positive thinking and affirmations to address your negative thoughts?
- How can you use positive thoughts and words to encourage others?
- What did you like about creating your Positive Thinking Sunshine?
- What was challenging about this activity?
- What did you learn from completing this activity?

Positive Thinking Sunshine Handout

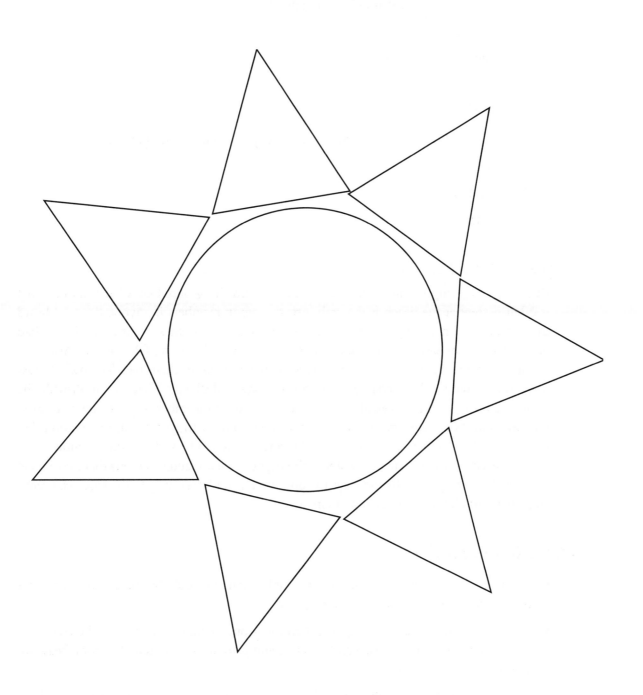

July
I'M FEELING CRABBY (SUMMER)

Purpose of the activity

- To identify triggers for frustration and anger
- To learn positive coping skills
- To promote self-awareness

Materials needed

- Copies of the I'm Feeling Crabby Handout (copied on heavy-weight paper)
- Red paint
- Paint brushes
- Pens, pencils

Description of the activity

Begin by discussing summertime and the beach with the group. One of the animals that is often present at the beach is the crab. Ask the group members if anyone has ever heard the expression "I'm feeling crabby." This is often used to describe someone who is in a bad mood, grumpy, or easily upset. Ask the participants if they have ever felt this way. Ask them to identify some triggers, events, or situations that may make them feel "crabby." Discuss ways to cope with feeling "crabby" and positive ways to deal with a bad mood. Provide the group members with the needed supplies. Ask each group member to paint the crab using the red paint. When they finish painting, ask them to list a trigger, event, or situation that makes them feel "crabby" next to each of the crab's arms and legs. When they complete this part of the activity, ask them to talk about the triggers, events, and situations that make them feel "crabby." As a group, discuss ways to cope and respond positively to the triggers, events, and situations identified by each participant.

Variations of the activity

- If you are short on time, the I'm Feeling Crabby Handout could be copied onto red paper or colored with red marker instead of paint.

- If you have more time in your group, then the group members can cut out the crab from the handout, trace it on to watercolor paper, and paint it using watercolors for a beautiful project.

- Instead of painting or coloring with markers, group members could make a collage of images, words, and drawings inside the crab to represent the triggers, events, and situations that make them feel "crabby."

- This activity works well paired with the Happy as a Clam activity (see next activity) for a short series on emotions, feelings, and coping skills.

- The I'm Feeling Crabby activity also works well in individual sessions.

Discussion questions

- What are some animals associated with summer and the beach?

- What does the expression "I'm feeling crabby" mean?

- Describe a time when you felt "crabby."

- How did you handle feeling "crabby?"

- Why is it not okay to take out our frustration and bad mood on others when we are feeling "crabby?"

- How does it feel when someone takes their frustration or bad mood out on you when they are feeling "crabby?"

- If you know that you are going to have to deal with a trigger or be in a situation that tends to put you in a bad mood or make you feel "crabby," how can you prepare beforehand to cope and prevent yourself from becoming angry or frustrated?

- What are some strategies that you use to cope when you are frustrated, in a bad mood, or feeling "crabby?"

- What is one new coping strategy that you can use to address each of the triggers, events, or situations that you identified on your I'm Feeling Crabby painting?

- What did you like about completing this activity?

- What was challenging about completing this activity?

- What did you learn from completing this activity?

I'm Feeling Crabby Handout

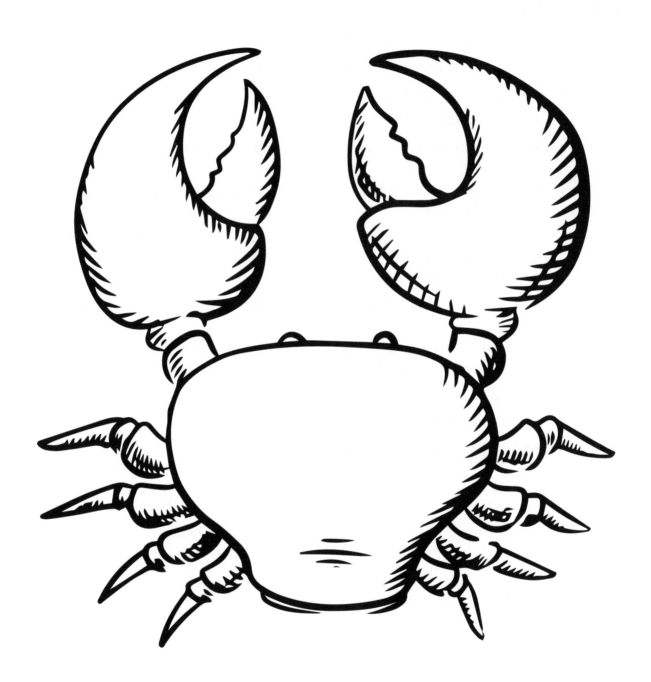

HAPPY AS A CLAM

Purpose of the activity

- To discuss happiness and ways to promote more happiness and joy

- To increase self-awareness and develop positive self-concept

- To identify healthy hobbies, leisure activities, and other outlets for enjoyment

Materials needed

- Copies of the Happy as a Clam Handout (copied on heavy-weight paper)

- Assorted colors of paint

- Paint brushes

- Pencils, pens, colored pencils

Description of the activity

Begin by discussing summer and the beach with the group members. If you have already completed the I'm Feeling Crabby activity (see previous activity) with group, review the information from this. Ask the group members if they have ever heard the expression "happy as a clam," used to describe a person who is very happy and content at the present moment. Ask the group to think of some situations and activities that make them feel as "happy as a clam." Examples might include spending time with friends, playing video games, drawing, or reading. These are just ideas to get the group members started in thinking about activities and experiences that bring them enjoyment and contentment. Distribute the needed materials to the group members. Ask each group member to paint his or her clam. As it dries, continue to discuss the importance of self-care and taking time to engage in leisure activities that bring enjoyment. When the Happy as a Clam paintings have dried, ask the group members to write words and phrases around their clam painting to represent activities, hobbies, events, and situations that bring them happiness and enjoyment. After they finish this part of the activity, ask them to share some of the things that they included on their clams.

Variations of the activity

- If you are short on time, the Happy as a Clam Handout could be colored using markers, crayons, or colored pencils instead of painting it.

- If you have more time in your group, the clam could be cut out and traced onto watercolor paper and painted using watercolor paint for a beautiful project.

- As an alternative, the group members could make a collage inside their clam using images, words, and drawings to represent the activities, hobbies, events, and situations that bring them happiness and enjoyment.

- The Happy as a Clam activity works well paired with the I'm Feeling Crabby activity (see previous activity) as a short series on feelings, emotions, and coping skills.
- This also works well as an activity for individual sessions.

Discussion questions

- What is your favorite thing about summertime?
- What are some animals associated with the beach?
- What does the expression "happy as a clam" mean?
- What does it mean to be happy?
- What does it mean to be content?
- What are some hobbies or activities that make you feel as "happy as a clam?"
- What are some situations or events that make you feel as "happy as a clam?"
- Why is it important to be self-aware and know the things that make us happy?
- What does the term "self-care" mean? What are some ways that we can take care of ourselves and stay healthy physically, emotionally, and mentally?
- How can you create more time in your life for self-care and for activities that bring you enjoyment and happiness?
- Describe a time when you felt happy and content.
- What did you like about completing this activity?
- What was challenging about completing this activity?
- What did you learn from completing this activity?

Happy as a Clam Handout

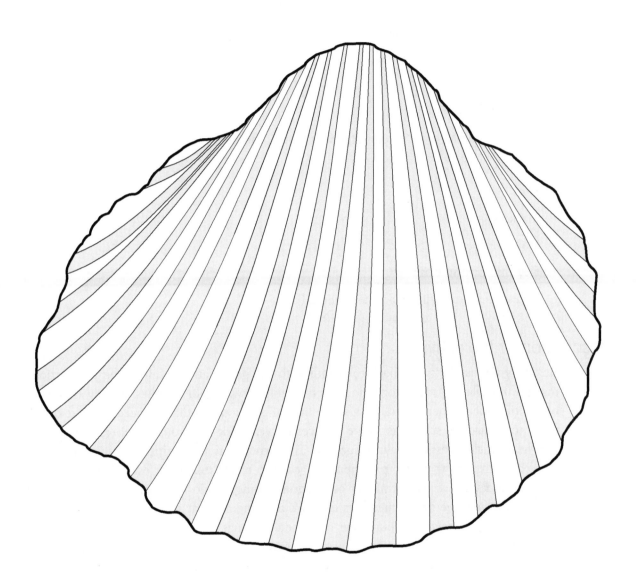

August
KEYS TO SUCCESS (PREPARING FOR GOING BACK TO SCHOOL)

Purpose of the activity

- To develop skills for goal setting, decision making, and organization
- To promote positive thinking
- To encourage self-awareness

Materials needed

- Copies of the Keys to Success Handout (copied on heavy-weight paper)
- Scissors
- Pens
- Markers
- Hole puncher
- Key ring or ring clasp
- Access to a laminating machine (optional)

Description of the activity

Begin by discussing going back to school with the group and the all of the preparations that go into getting ready for school such buying new school supplies, getting uniforms, or meeting the teachers. Next, discuss the mental preparations that we need to make to get ready to go back to school and have a successful year. Ask the group members if they have ever heard the expression "keys to success." This expression means tips for success or secrets to success. Explain that each participant is going to create his or her own Keys to Success key ring today to use as a reminder of important things to do to be successful in the new school year. Ask the group members to think of some areas at school that they struggled with during the previous school year or some areas that they would like to improve this school year. Examples might include completing homework daily, asking for help with assignments when needed, using conflict resolution skills to avoid fights, coming to class with the right materials, etc. Assist the group members in developing their personal keys to success as needed. Once all of them have identified their keys to success for the new school year, distribute the needed supplies. Ask group members to write one of their keys to success on each of the keys on the Keys to Success Handout. Next, they can color and decorate their keys, and cut them out and laminate them (if possible). After the keys have been cut out and laminated, assist the group members in punching holes in the top of each key and then placing them on the key ring or ring clasp. Discuss ways to use the Keys to Success as a reminders and tips for things to do each day for a successful school year.

Variations of the activity

- A great place for the group members to keep their Keys to Success is attached to the rings of a three-ring binder that is frequently used so that the keys will be frequently viewed and easily accessible.

- This also works well as an activity for an individual session.

- Keys to Success can be created for more specific areas or settings, if desired. For example, the group members could create Keys to Success for Resolving Conflicts, Keys to Success for Organization, Keys to Success for Managing Anger, Keys to Success for Home, Keys to Success for Group Meetings, etc.

Discussion questions

- What are your thoughts and feelings about going back to school?

- What kind of things do you have to do to get ready to go back to school?

- How can you prepare mentally for the new school year?

- What is an area that you would like to improve this school year?

- What does it mean to be successful?

- How will you know if you are successful in meeting your goals for the new school year?

- What does the expression "keys to success" mean?

- What will be some of your Keys to Success as you get ready to go back to school this year?

- Why is it important to set goals and think about ways to be successful in different areas at school?

- What are some of your personal Keys to Success that you have identified and listed on your keys?

- What are some ways that you can apply your Keys to Success in different areas at school?

- Where will you keep your Keys to Success so that you can refer to them frequently as reminders for positive tips and behaviors at school?

- How can you use or adapt your Keys to Success for other settings such as home or after-school activities?

- What did you like about completing this activity?

- What was challenging about completing this activity?

- What did you learn from completing this activity?

Keys to Success Handout

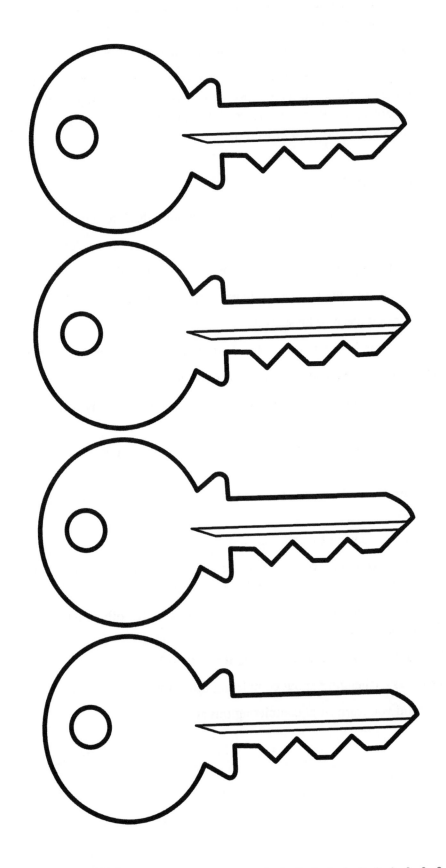

KICKING OFF THE NEW SCHOOL YEAR WITH GOOD BEHAVIOR (BACK TO SCHOOL)

Purpose of the activity

- To identify and learn acceptable rules and behaviors for school settings
- To promote positive social skills
- To encourage self-awareness

Materials needed

- Copies of the Kicking Off the New School Year with Good Behavior Handout
- Markers, pens, colored pencils
- Scissors

Description of the activity

This activity is a good way to introduce classroom rules or behavioral expectations at the beginning of the school year. Start by reviewing the rules and expectations with the group. Give examples of situations and ask group members to state the appropriate rule or behavioral response for the situation. Provide scenarios and ask group members to role play how to respond correctly to each scenario based on the rules or behavioral expectations. Next, provide the group members with the needed supplies. Explain to them that they are going to create a soccer ball with the rules or behavioral expectations listed on it as a reminder to be "Kicking Off the New School Year with Good Behavior." Ask the participants to list the rules or behavior expectations on the white parts of the soccer ball on the handout. When this is complete, ask them to cut out their soccer balls. Review the rules and ask group members to explain the rules in their own words.

Variations of the activity

- The completed soccer balls could slide in the cover of a three-ring binder or in a sheet protector inside a binder for frequent viewing. Refer to the soccer balls frequently as a reminder of rules and behavioral expectations for group members.
- Group members can also create their own soccer balls using white paper plates and black construction paper. They can cut pentagon shapes out of the black construction paper and glue them to the white paper plate. The rules and behavioral expectations can then be written on the white spaces on the paper plate.
- The completed soccer balls make a fun display for the beginning of the school year with the heading "We're Kicking Off the School Year with Good Behavior."

Discussion questions

- How do you feel about rules and expectations?

- What are some reasons that we need rules and expectations?

- What might happen if there were no rules or expectations?

- What are some of the positive things that might happen as a result of following the rules and expectations?

- What happens if you do not follow the rules and expectations?

- Explain the rules to me in your own words.

- Give an example of how the rules might apply to a real-life situation.

- Why is it important to start the school year off by following the rules and expectations?

- Where will you keep your Kicking Off the New School Year with Good Behavior soccer ball so that you will be reminded frequently of the rules and expectations?

- What did you like about this activity?

- What was challenging about this activity?

- What did you learn from this activity?

Kicking Off the New School Year with Good Behavior Handout

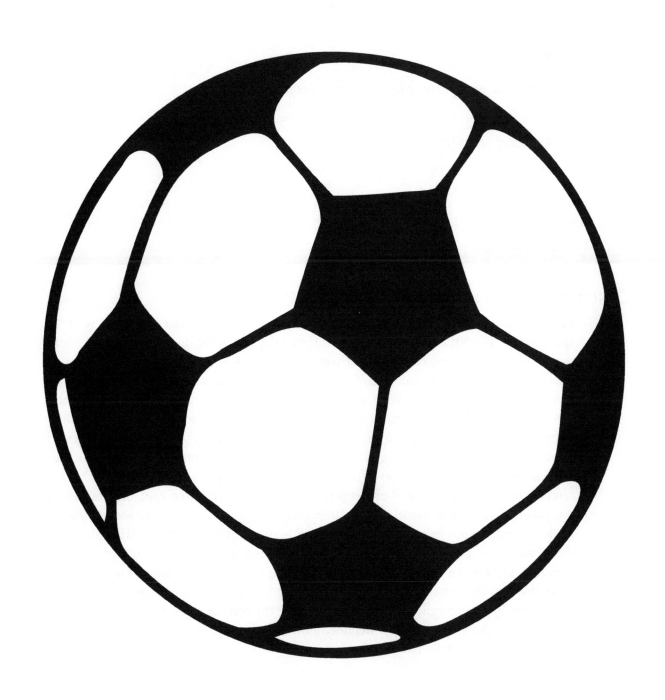

September
AN APPLE A DAY (FALL)

Purpose of the activity

- To understand the importance of self-care
- To promote self-awareness and positive self-concept
- To learn healthy ways to care for physical, mental, and emotional health

Materials needed

- Large piece of paper (one for each group member)
- Red paint
- Styrofoam plates (or trays for paint)
- Pens, markers
- Apples
- Knife (to cut apples in half)
- Cutting board

Description of the activity

Begin by asking the group if anyone has ever heard the expression that starts with "An apple a day." The whole expression is "An apple a day keeps the doctor away." This means that by eating apples and taking care of yourself you will stay healthy and not need to see a doctor. Discuss the importance of self-care with the group and assist the group members in identifying ways to take care of their physical, mental, and emotional health. Ask them to identify some of the reasons that it is important to take care of ourselves and stay healthy. Distribute paper, plates with red paint and half an apple to each group member. Ask each group member to dip their apple half in the red paint and then press it down on the sheet of paper to make the impression of an apple. Ask the group members to repeat this step several times. Each group member needs to have at least eight to ten apple impressions on the paper. These can be done in any pattern that the group member chooses. While the apple impressions dry, help the group to identify ways that they can stay healthy physically, emotionally, and mentally. Examples might include exercising, drinking more water, keeping a journal, using anger management strategies. When the apple impressions are dry, ask the group members to write one of the ways that they identified to stay healthy on or around each of the apple impressions on their paper using the pens or markers. Ask them to share the strategies and ways that they identified how to stay healthy and how they will utilize these strategies on a daily basis.

Variations of the activity

- If you are short on time for the session, you could have apple shapes cut out of red construction paper and ready to glue to the paper instead of using the apple halves and red paint.

- This also works well as an individual activity.

- This activity makes a great display for bulletin boards or group meeting spaces, using the heading "We're Staying Healthy with an Apple a Day."

- The activity could also be completed as a group mural. A large tree can be painted on the mural paper and then the group members can draw or paint apples on the tree. They can then write the ways that they will stay healthy physically, mentally, and emotionally around the apples on the tree.

- After completing the activity, consider serving a special apple snack to the group. Making caramel apples is a fun way to coordinate with the activity theme.

Discussion questions

- What does the expression "An apple a day keeps the doctor away" mean?

- Why is it important to take care of ourselves?

- What are some ways to stay physically healthy?

- What are some ways to stay emotionally healthy?

- What are some ways to stay mentally healthy?

- What are some reasons that we have to focus on all three areas of health (physical, mental, and emotional)?

- What might happen if we only focused on one of the areas (physical, mental, or emotional)?

- How does it impact us if we are not taking care of ourselves in one of the three areas?

- How does it impact the people around us if we are not taking care of ourselves in one of the three areas?

- What are some of the ways that you identified to stay healthy in this activity?

- What changes will you have to make to become healthy in the different areas of your life?

- How will you implement the strategies that you identified in your An Apple a Day activity?

- What did you like about completing this activity?

- What was challenging about this activity?

- What did you learn from completing this activity?

NATURE SCAVENGER HUNT (FALL)

Purpose of the activity

- To develop and practice following directions
- To encourage positive social skills
- To promote communication skills

Materials needed

- Copies of the Nature Scavenger Hunt Handouts 1 and 2
- Brown paper bags (lunch size)
- Access to outdoor location
- Special snacks to reward those who complete the activity
- Four prizes (for winning teams)

Description of the activity

Begin by telling the group that they are going to participate in a Nature Scavenger Hunt today. Explain that the group members will be divided into pairs to complete the scavenger hunt. The partners in each pair will have to work together because each person will have a list of different items to find. In order to complete the scavenger hunt and earn the reward, the pairs will have to find all of the items on both lists. Explain that they must work together and cannot simply go and find the items on their own list to complete the scavenger hunt. Consider pairing group members who might not usually choose to work together in order to allow new relationships to be built and new opportunities to practice social skills. Distribute paper bags to all of the group members. Explain that everyone who completes the activity will earn a reward, but special rewards will be given to the team that does the best job working together and the team that finishes the scavenger hunt first with the correct items from the handouts. Give one copy of the Nature Scavenger Hunt Handout 1 to one member of each team and give one copy of the Nature Scavenger Hunt Handout 2 to the other member. Observe the group members as they complete the activity to see if there are any issues that will need to be discussed once the activity is complete. After the Nature Scavenger Hunt is done, discuss the activity with the group. Give prizes to the team that finished first and the team that did the best job working together. Give a special snack to all the group members who completed the hunt.

Variations of the activity

- This Nature Scavenger Hunt is based around items found outside during the fall. It could be changed for spring, summer, or winter, or customized for the area where you live.
- Scavenger hunts are a fun way to encourage skills in following directions. Instead of finding items that are readily available outside, you could hide items and write clues

that require following directions in order to find them. This is a fun way to complete a scavenger hunt on holidays. For example, on Valentine's Day, you could hide red paper hearts and then write clues with directions that lead to each heart.

Discussion questions

- What is a scavenger hunt?
- What skills will you have to use to win the scavenger hunt?
- What will happen if you and your partner do not work together?
- What does it mean to cooperate and work as a team?
- How can you be a team player and work with your partner?
- What will happen if you do not follow directions or do not get the items listed on your Nature Scavenger Hunt Handout?

After the hunt:

- How well did you and your partner work as a team?
- How well did you follow directions? Did you get the items listed on your handout?
- What can you do to improve your skills in following directions?
- Were the any issues with working with your partner while completing the activity? If so, please explain.
- What can you do to be more of a team player in the future?
- What did you like about this activity?
- What was challenging about this activity?
- What did you learn from completing this activity?

Nature Scavenger Hunt Handout 1

Please find the following items:

☐   One brown leaf

☐   One small stick

☐   Three smooth rocks

☐   Two blades of grass

☐   One small acorn

☐   Two yellow leaves

Nature Scavenger Hunt Handout 2

Please find the following items:

- [ ] One medium size stick

- [ ] One red leaf

- [ ] One large rock

- [ ] Three small stones

- [ ] One pinecone

- [ ] Two brown leaves

October

WHAT A TANGLED WEB WE WEAVE (HALLOWEEN/FALL)

Purpose of the activity

- To discuss honesty and the importance of telling the truth
- To encourage self-awareness and positive self-concept
- To promote social skills

Materials needed

- Paper plates
- Scissors
- Black paint, markers, crayons
- White paint marker
- Paint brushes
- Hole punches
- Yarn
- Glue sticks
- Glitter

Description of the activity

Begin by asking the group members if they have ever heard the expression "What a tangled web we weave when first we practice to deceive." Explain that this expression means that when we tell a lie, we have to continue to tell more lies and "weave a tangled web" to keep others believing the lie. Discuss the importance of honesty and telling the truth with the group. Discuss the consequences of telling lies with the group members and explain that they are going to create a "tangled web" today as a visual reminder of the lesson. Distribute the needed supplies. First, ask each individual to cut out the center of the paper plate (discard this or save it for a later project) while leaving the outer part intact. Next, ask the group members to punch holes all the way around the inside of the paper plate. Depending on the timeframe, group members can then paint the plate black or color it black using a black marker or crayon to complete the activity more quickly. Provide each individual with a long piece of yarn and ask them to thread the yarn through the holes which are across from each other in the paper plate, to create the pattern of a spider web. Begin by knotting one end of the piece of yarn on the outside of one of the holes. After the yarn has been threaded through all of the holes, pull it tight, tie a knot on the outside of the last hole, and cut off any excess. If desired, the group members can use the glue stick to glue all around the paper plate and then sprinkle it with the glitter. A hole can also be punched at the top of the plate and tied with yarn so that the What a Tangled Web We Weave paper plates could become a hanging display. On the back of the paper plate, the group members could write "What a tangled web we weave when first we practice to deceive" in white paint marker if desired. Finish by discussing real-life scenarios, how to handle the scenarios, and what the outcome might be of telling the truth or a lie.

Variations of the activity

- These spider web paper plates make a fun display. The heading could be "We are Truthful… No Tangled Webs to Weave for Us!"

- Consider having a party with fun snacks for Halloween after completing the activity. You could make "spiders" by sticking pretzel sticks in the side of a marshmallow and using mini M&Ms for the eyes.

Discussion questions

- What does the expression "What a tangled web we weave when first we practice to deceive" mean?

- How do we "weave a tangled web" when we tell a lie?

- What happens when you have to tell a second lie to cover up the first lie?

- How do you feel when you tell a lie?

- What are some of the consequences of telling a lie?

- Why is it important to tell the truth?

- What are some of the benefits of being honest and telling the truth?

- What does it mean to be honest?

- What situations might make you feel tempted to lie instead of tell the truth?

- Why do you think people choose to tell lies instead of the truth?

- How would you feel if you found out that one of your friends told you a lie?

- What should you do if telling the truth might hurt someone's feelings?

- What should you do if telling the truth might get you or a friend in trouble?

- How can you become trustworthy again if you have told lies before?

- What are some of the advantages of being a truthful and honest person?

- Is it ever okay to tell a lie? Explain your answer.

- What does the expression "The truth will set you free" mean? Do you agree with this? Explain your answer.

- What can you do to become a more honest and truthful person?

- What did you like about this activity?

- What was challenging about this activity?

- What did you learn from participating in this activity?

MELTING AWAY OUR ANGER MINI PUMPKINS (HALLOWEEN/FALL)

Purpose of the activity

- To discuss anger management and de-escalation strategies
- To encourage self-awareness
- To promote conflict resolution skills and social skills

Materials needed

- Mini pumpkins (one per group member)
- White spray paint
- Assorted colors of crayons (paper removed and cut in half)
- Tacky glue
- Hair dryer
- Wax paper or other covering to protect table surface

Description of the activity

In advance of the group, spray paint mini pumpkins white and allow them to dry, or purchase white mini pumpkins if available. Begin by discussing anger management and de-escalation techniques with the group. Discuss some ways to let anger "melt away." Letting go of our anger can be a positive and beautiful process. Assist the group members with identifying different ways to manage their anger. Distribute the needed supplies to the group members. Place a piece of wax paper underneath each pumpkin. Ask each group member to glue the assorted colors of crayon halves around the stem of the pumpkin. They should be able to fit between 10 and 15 crayon halves around the top of the pumpkin. Once they have glued the crayon halves, use the hairdryer to heat the crayons on the mini pumpkins until they melt and drip down the side of the pumpkin. Allow this to dry and for the melted crayons to harden on side of the pumpkin. Discuss how beautiful the mini pumpkins are now that the crayons have melted and added color all around the pumpkins. Explain that it is the same way with anger. As we let go of anger, we are able to enjoy the beauty around us. Discuss other benefits of anger management with the group members. Allow them to take their completed mini pumpkins home with them as a reminder to let their anger melt away.

Variations of the activity

- This activity could also be completed during any season using a white canvas or white candle. Follow the same procedure described above to attach the crayons to the canvas or candle using tacky glue and then heat with a hair dryer until the crayons melt down the side of the canvas or candle.

- Consider having a fun party to celebrate fall after completing the activity. The group members could make pumpkin rice krispie treats by coloring the rice krispie treat batter orange using food coloring, shaping it into round balls, and inserting a tootsie roll in the top center to serve as the pumpkin stem.

Discussion questions

- What does it mean to be angry?

- Describe a time when you felt angry. How did you feel?

- What are some observable signs that you are angry?

- How can you tell if someone else is angry?

- What are some positive ways to manage your anger?

- What does it mean to let your anger "melt away?"

- What are some different ways that you can let your anger "melt away?"

- How can it be a positive and beautiful process to let your anger "melt away?"

- How would you describe the mini pumpkins once the crayons melted?

- Were the pumpkins more beautiful when they were solid white or once they were covered with the different colors of melted crayons? Explain your answer.

- How are we more able to enjoy the beauty around us when we let our anger "melt away?"

- What is one new strategy that you can use to let your anger "melt away?"

- What do you think will be different if you are not as angry?

- What did you like about completing this activity?

- What was challenging about this activity?

- What did you learn from participating in this activity?

November
LETTING GO OF NEGATIVITY LEAF ART (FALL)
Purpose of the activity

- To promote positive thinking skills

- To encourage self-awareness and positive self-concept

- To encourage creativity and self-expression

Materials needed

- Leaves

- Tacky glue

- Pens, colored pencils, markers

- White paper (heavy weight, such as cardstock)

Description of the activity

Discuss some of the events that occur during the fall that can be observed outdoors. Some examples might be cooler temperatures, pumpkins and other fall crops ready for harvest, and leaves changing color and falling down from the trees. Discuss with the group that the trees have to "let go" of the old and dead leaves and let them fall away so that new leaves can grow when the spring comes. Explain that this concept can also be applied to our lives and the way we think. At times, we have to "let go" of negative thoughts and ways of thinking and doing things in order to move forward and grow. Assist the group in identifying some negative thoughts, patterns, or behaviors that they want to let go of so that new thoughts and behaviors can grow and replace them. Help them to identify some of these new behaviors and thoughts that they would like to see grow in their lives. Explain that they are going to create Letting Go of Negativity Leaf Art to help them remember to let go, let negativity fall away, and make room for the new behaviors and thoughts to grow, just like trees do with their leaves in the fall.

If time allows, take the group members outside to select their own leaves. Flat leaves work best for this activity. If you do not have time for this, gather an assortment of leaves in different sizes and colors in advance for the group members to choose from. Provide them with the other needed supplies. Ask them to glue their leaf anywhere they like on their paper. Next, ask them to use the writing and drawing supplies to turn the leaf into something new. The possibilities are endless. They might choose to turn the leaf into a drawing of an animal, a car, a person, an abstract design, etc. When all of the group members have completed their project, discuss each individuals' creation from the leaves. Review the earlier discussion and remind them that when we let go of negative thoughts and behaviors, we make room for new and positive things to emerge in our lives.

Variations of the activity

- This also works well as an individual activity.

- This activity could be incorporate into a science class during the fall.

- The completed leaf art projects make a fun display with the heading "Letting Go of Negativity Leaf Art."

- Instead of creating new art from leaves, the group could write the thoughts or behaviors that they want to "let go" of on different leaves using paint markers and then take the leaves outside and let them "fall away" with all of the other leaves that are falling down from trees.

Discussion questions

- What are some of the changes that happen outside during the fall season?

- What happens to the leaves on the trees during the fall?

- What would happen to trees if the dead leaves did not fall away and make room for new leaves to grow when spring comes each year?

- What are some things that people need to let go of in order to grow and learn new ways of thinking and behaving?

- What happens if we do not let go of negative thoughts and ways of behaving in our lives?

- What are some negative thoughts, patterns, or behaviors that you need to let go of in order to grow in a positive way?

- What is stopping you from letting go of these negative thoughts and behaviors?

- What changes would you have to make in order to let go of the negative thoughts and behaviors?

- How have negative thoughts and behaviors held you back from growing in positive ways?

- What positive thoughts and behaviors do you want to see grow in your life?

- What did you create with your leaf on your Letting Go of Negativity Leaf Art activity?

- How does your Letting Go of Negativity Leaf Art represent the positive growth and change that can come from "letting go" of negativity and other thoughts and behaviors that may be holding you back in life?

- Where will you display your leaf art so that you will be reminded to let go of negativity and allow positive thoughts and behaviors to grow in your life?

- What did you like about this activity?

- What was challenging about this activity?

- What did you learn from this activity?

THANKFULNESS KITS (THANKSGIVING)

Purpose of the activity

- To promote the expression of gratitude and thankfulness
- To encourage positive thinking
- To develop social skills

Materials needed

- Pencil box, empty travel wipes container (hard plastic), or other similar sized container with a lid (one per group member)
- Sticky notes or small index cards
- Markers, pens, colored pencils
- Thank-you cards and envelopes (cards could be store bought or handmade)
- Stamps

Description of the activity

Begin by discussing gratitude and the importance of being thankful with the group. Discuss some of the reasons why it is important to be thankful for the blessings and good things in our lives. Talk about ways to show others that we are thankful for them and reasons why it is important to let others know we appreciate them. While it is important to express thankfulness and gratitude at Thanksgiving, it is also important to express thankfulness and gratitude throughout the year. Explain to the group members that they are going to create Thankfulness Kits to make expressing gratitude a more frequent part of their life. Distribute all of the materials to the group members. Ask them to place a pad of sticky notes in their container. The sticky notes are a quick place to jot down a few things that they are thankful for each day. Next, the group members can add the thank-you notes to their Thankfulness Kit. If time allows, they could also create their own handmade thank-you notes. Ask the participants to think of one person in their life who is a positive influence and a blessing to them. Ask them to write a thank-you note to this person, letting him or her know how much he or she is appreciated. Provide stamps for mailing the thank-you notes if necessary. Ask the group members to make a commitment to either write one thank-you note or show gratitude in another meaningful way to someone who is making a difference in their lives each week.

Variations of the activity

- If desired, the container could be covered using fabric (glued on with tacky glue) and then trimmed with piping to make the Thankfulness Kit even more special.
- If your group meets daily, consider having Thankful Thursdays each week. At the beginning of the group session on Thursday, the group members can use their Thankfulness Kits to write down a few things they are thankful for that week and then write a thank-you note to someone meaningful to them.

Discussion questions

- Why do we celebrate Thanksgiving?

- What does it mean to be thankful?

- What does the word "gratitude" mean?

- What are some reasons we should be thankful for all the good things in our lives?

- Why should we let others know that we are thankful for them?

- What are some meaningful ways to show others that we are grateful for them?

- How do you feel when others tell you that they are thankful for you?

- What happens when we take the good things in our lives for granted or become unappreciative of the good things we have?

- How can writing down the things that we are thankful for each day keep us focused on positive things?

- Have you ever received a thank-you note from someone? If so, how did it make you feel?

- How do you feel when someone tells you thank you or notices something nice that you have done?

- What are some ways that we can remain grateful and thankful throughout the year?

- How can you make thankfulness and focusing on the positives a habit in your life?

- Can you name one meaningful person in your life who you can take the time to write a thank-you note to this week?

- How can we use the Thankfulness Kits in group sessions to keep focused on gratitude and positive things?

- What did you like about creating the Thankfulness Kits?

- What will be challenging about continuing to use the Thankfulness Kits?

- What did you learn from participating in this activity?

December

WE'RE LETTING OUR LIGHTS SHINE (CHRISTMAS)

Purpose of the activity

- To identify ways to serve others

- To promote social skills

- To encourage self-awareness and positive self-concept

Materials needed

- Copies of the We're Letting Our Lights Shine Handout (copied on card stock or heavy-weight paper)

- Markers, pens, crayons

- Scissors

- Hole puncher

- Ribbon, string, yarn

Description of the activity

Begin by discussing some of the signs and symbols of Christmas. Explain that Christmas lights are one of the signs of the Christmas season. People put lights on their houses and Christmas trees to add light in the darkness. Discuss how each group member can also be a "light" to others in the darkness during the Christmas season and throughout the year. Assist the group members in identifying ways that they can serve others and be a "light" in the lives of others. When we help others and show concern for others, our lights are shining. Distribute the needed supplies to the group members. Ask them to write one way they are going to let their lights shine by helping others this Christmas season on the light on the We're Letting Our Lights Shine Handout. They can then color and decorate their light using the markers and crayons. Next, the group members can cut out their Christmas light and punch a hole in the top of it. The lights can be strung together and connected using the ribbon, yarn, or string. Follow up with the group members throughout the Christmas season and ask them to identify ways that they are helping others and letting their lights shine. Remind them that it is easy to become focused on ourselves and all the busyness of the season, but it is important to take time to help others and give to those in need around us.

Variations of the activity

- This activity makes a great display for bulletin boards and group meeting areas with the heading "We're Letting Our Lights Shine."

- Consider having the group members come up with a group project that will serve others during the Christmas season and all let their "lights shine together."

- If your group meets regularly, keep copies of the We're Letting Our Lights Shine Handout available. Each time a group member does something kind or helps others during the Christmas season, ask him or her to write down what he or she did on the handout, cut out the light, and add it to the string of lights.

Discussion questions

- What are some of the signs and symbols of the Christmas season?

- What are some of the reasons why people put up Christmas lights?

- How do Christmas lights bring light to the darkness?

- What are some ways that you can be a "light" in the darkness for others?

- How can you help those around you during the Christmas season?

- What is one way that you can let your light shine this Christmas season?

- Why should we take time to help others?

- What are some of the things that might keep us from helping others and letting our lights shine?

- Why is it easy to become focused on ourselves during the Christmas season?

- How can you shift your focus to letting your light shine for others?

- What are some of the positive things that could happen as a result of letting your light shine for others?

- How can we work together as a group to let our lights shine?

- What did you like about this activity?

- What do you think will be a challenge as you are letting your light shine?

- What did you learn from completing this activity?

We're Letting Our Lights Shine Handout

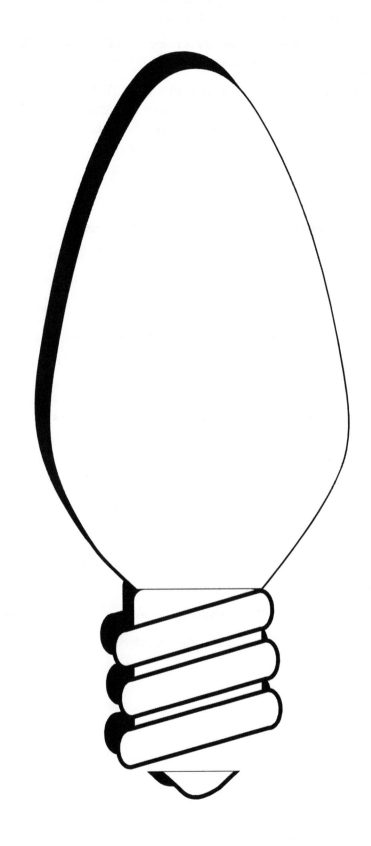

SALT DOUGH ORNAMENTS TO SHARE (CHRISTMAS)

Purpose of the activity

- To develop positive social skills
- To encourage empathy and kindness to others
- To promote skills in following directions

Materials needed

- All-purpose flour (four cups)
- Salt (one cup)
- Water (approximately one-and-a-half cups)
- Cinnamon (optional)
- Rolling pin
- Plastic drinking straws
- Ribbon
- Christmas cookie cutters (Christmas trees, candy canes, etc.)
- Wax paper
- Baking sheet
- Access to an oven
- Acrylic paint (optional)
- Paint brushes (optional)
- Mod Podge Sealer Spray
- Copies of the Salt Dough Ornaments to Share Handout
- Scissors
- Hole puncher

Description of the activity

Begin by asking the group to discuss some of the traditions associated with Christmas, such as giving gifts to others. Ask the group members if it is better to give than to receive. Discuss the benefits of giving to others. Explain to the group that they are going to create salt dough ornaments to share with others this Christmas season.

Begin by preheating the oven to 300 degrees. Combine the flour, salt, and water to create a dough. If desired, add cinnamon (a few tablespoons) to give the dough a pleasant scent. Knead the dough a few times and then roll it out using a rolling pin to about a half-inch thickness. Using Christmas cookie cutters, cut the dough into desired shapes. Make a hole at the top of each ornament with a plastic drinking straw (the ribbon to hang the ornament will be threaded through this hole). Bake at 300 degrees on a baking sheet lined with wax paper for approximately 1 hour 15 minutes to 1 hour 30 minutes. Allow to cool. If desired, paint the shapes with acrylic paint and seal with Mod Podge or another sealant. Cover the workspace with wax paper to protect it. When dry, thread with ribbon and tie. Cut gift tags out from the Salt Dough Ornaments to Share Handout, punch a hole in each tag, and attach them with ribbon to the ornaments. If you do not have access to an oven at the group location, you can roll out the dough, cut shapes, place them on cookie sheets, take the ornaments home to bake, and return them the next day.

Assist the group members in identifying individuals to give the salt dough ornaments to as gifts. Ask them to think of someone who might be feeling sad during the holiday season and might need to be cheered up. Remind the group members that it is important to take time to give to others. If possible, the group could take a field trip to a local nursing home to deliver the ornaments to the residents.

Variations of the activity

- Instead of paint, you can also use food coloring to color the dough. Make the dough several shades darker with the food coloring than you would like it to be because it will lighten as it bakes.

- For Valentine's Day, the group could make hearts to paint and then give to others.

- The salt dough ornaments also make great gifts for Mother's Day or Father's Day. Instead of cutting shapes using cookie cutters, the group members can make prints of their hands in the dough and give the handprint as a gift on these days.

- During the summer time, the group could make salt dough sunshine ornaments to give to others. You could make little gift tags to attach that say "Just bringing you a little sunshine to brighten your day."

Discussion questions

- What are some traditions that you associate with Christmas and the holiday season?

- Describe the tradition of giving gifts at Christmas.

- Is it better to give or to receive? Please explain your answer.

- What are the benefits of giving to others?

- Why is it important to give to others?

- During the holiday season when everyone is very busy, why is it important to take time to give to those in need?

- How can a small gift lift someone's spirits?

- Describe the best gift you ever received.

- Describe the best gift you ever gave to someone else.

- What makes a handmade gift special?

- Who in your life might benefit from receiving a salt dough ornament to lift their spirits?

- Sometimes people feel sad during the holiday season. What are some ways to cope if you feel sad at this time?

- What did you enjoy about this activity?

- What was challenging about this activity?

- What did you learn from this activity?

Salt Dough Ornament to Share Handout

Please enjoy this salt dough ornament! Made especially for you by_____	Please enjoy this salt dough ornament! Made especially for you by_____
Please enjoy this salt dough ornament! Made especially for you by_____	Please enjoy this salt dough ornament! Made especially for you by_____
Please enjoy this salt dough ornament! Made especially for you by_____	Please enjoy this salt dough ornament! Made especially for you by_____
Please enjoy this salt dough ornament! Made especially for you by_____	Please enjoy this salt dough ornament! Made especially for you by_____
Please enjoy this salt dough ornament! Made especially for you by_____	Please enjoy this salt dough ornament! Made especially for you by_____

OVERVIEW OF MY YEAR (NEW YEAR'S EVE)

Purpose of the activity

- To promote self-awareness and positive self-concept
- To develop positive thinking skills and goal-setting skills
- To identify positive aspects of the year and goals or areas for improvement in the new year

Materials needed

- Copies of the Overview of My Year Handout
- Pens, pencils, markers

Description of the activity

Begin by discussing New Year's Eve with the group. New Year's Eve is a time for reflection and for spending time reviewing the positive things that happened in the past year as well as identifying areas for improvement in the coming year. Distribute copies of the Overview of My Year Handout and writing supplies. Ask the group members to spend a few minutes thinking about the items on the handout and writing in their responses. The group members can also decorate their handouts using the markers. When they have completed the handouts, discuss each individual's responses. Assist the group members in developing goals for the areas of improvement that they identified on their handouts. Discuss each group member's positive experiences of the past year and ways to continue to stay on the right path in these areas.

Variations of the activity

- This activity could also be adapted to use at the end of the school year to reflect on and review the past year and develop positive goals for the next school year.
- This activity also works well for individual sessions.

Discussion questions

- What do you know about New Year's Eve?
- Why is it important to spend time reflecting on what went well over the past year and identifying areas for improvement for the coming year?
- What will happen if we don't ever take time to reflect on where we have come from and where we are going in life?
- Many people set new year's resolutions at this time of year. What is a new year's resolution?
- How do you feel about setting resolutions or goals?

- What might happen if we do not set any goals for ourselves?

- Tell me about the responses you included on your Overview of My Year Handout.

- What was the best thing that happened to you in the past year?

- How can you stay on the right path in the areas in which things have gone well during the past year?

- What are some areas in which you would like to improve in the new year?

- What is a specific goal that you can work toward in one of the areas that you would like to improve?

- How will you know if you have been successful in meeting your goal?

- What did you like about this activity?

- What was challenging about this activity?

- What did you learn from participating in this activity?

Overview of My Year (_____) Handout

Name: . . . . Age: . . . .

World events this year: . . . .

. . . .

Favorites:

Food: . . . . TV show: . . . .

Movie: . . . . Celebrity: . . . .

Music: . . . . Hobby: . . . .

Subject: . . . . Store: . . . .

Book: . . . . Sport: . . . .

Best thing that happened this year: . . . .

. . . .

Biggest change or challenge this year: . . . .

. . . .

Things that worked well this year that I want to continue: . . . .

. . . .

Goals for the new year: . . . .

. . . .

Changes I want to make in the new year: . . . .

. . . .

CHAPTER 5

Bibliotherapy Activities

STAND TALL, MOLLY LOU MELON BY PATTY LOVELL (AUTHOR) AND DAVID CATROW (ILLUSTRATOR)

Synopsis

Mollie Lou Melon has a way of turning her weaknesses into strengths with the encouragement and support of her grandmother, but when Mollie Lou Melon has to move to a new town away from her friends and grandmother, the school bully begins to tease her. Mollie Lou Melon copes with the teasing in a positive manner, makes a new friend in the process, and sends her grandmother a thank-you note telling her that all of her advice was correct.

Purpose of the activity

- To promote positive thinking skills
- To encourage self-awareness and positive self-concept
- To show appreciation and gratitude to others

Materials needed

- Copy of *Stand Tall, Molly Lou Melon*
- Copies of the Thumbprint Thank-You Note Handout
- Ink pad
- Heavy-weight paper or card stock paper
- Envelopes
- Pens, pencils, markers
- Copies of the Weaknesses to Strengths Handout

Description of the activity

Read the book (*Stand Tall, Molly Lou Melon*) with the participant. Discuss the book and some of its concepts, including positive thinking, turning weaknesses into strengths, coping with being bullied or teased, and showing appreciation to those who believe in us. Discuss the fact that everyone is unique with areas of strength and areas of weakness. However, our weaknesses can become strengths depending on how we view these areas. Discuss some of Molly Lou Melon's weaknesses that she turned into strengths and positive areas in her life. Discuss ways to show appreciation to those who believe in us and encourage us.

ACTIVITY 1: THUMBPRINT THANK-YOU NOTE

Provide the participants with the needed supplies. Explain that they are going to create a Thumbprint Thank-You Note because each person's thumbprint is unique, just as we are all unique with strengths and weaknesses. The Thumbprint Thank-You Note will be given to someone who has encouraged and believed in them. Assist the participants in placing their thumbs in the ink and then pressing their thumbprints down several times around the poem on their Thumbprint Thank-You Notes. Ask them to write a short note to the person thanking him or her for the specific ways he or she has made a difference in their life. The participants can also decorate the thank-you note and envelope. The Thumbprint Thank-You Note can then be given to the special people in their lives or you can provide stamps and assist with writing out the address and mailing the thank-you notes.

ACTIVITY 2: WEAKNESSES TO STRENGTHS

Discuss the ways that Molly Lou Melon turned things that others might perceive as "weaknesses" or "flaws" into strengths and special things about her. Provide the participants with copies of the Weaknesses to Strengths Handout and writing supplies. In the weaknesses column of the handout ask them to list a few things that they might consider weaknesses, that they do not like about themselves, or that others might tease them about. Next, help them to develop positive statements or ways that each perceived weakness could become an area of strength in their lives.

Variations of the activity

- If the participants struggle with negative thoughts, they could list of each of the positive statements and strengths that they identified on the Weaknesses to Strengths Handout on small cards that they could keep with them in a pocket, binder, or wallet to refer to frequently and promote positive thinking and coping skills

Discussion questions

- Please summarize the book (*Stand Tall, Molly Lou Melon*) we just read.
- What was your favorite part of the book?
- What was your least favorite part of the book?
- Is *Stand Tall, Molly Lou Melon* realistic? Please explain your answer.

- How does Molly Lou Melon use positive thinking skills?

- How does Molly Lou Melon turn things that some people might consider "weaknesses" or "flaws" into strengths or positive aspects of her life?

- How does Molly Lou Melon cope with being bullied and teased?

- How does the person who is teasing Molly Lou Melon end up becoming her friend?

- How does Molly Lou Melon show her appreciation for the support of her grandmother?

- What can you learn from Molly Lou Melon?

- How can you turn some of the things that you perceive as weaknesses into strengths or positive areas of your life?

- How can you cope in a positive way if you are teased or bullied?

- How can you show appreciation to those who believe in you and encourage you?

- Why is it important to write thank-you notes or show our appreciation to those who encourage us?

- How can you focus on positive thoughts and improve your positive thinking skills?

- How does it feel to take time to show appreciation and gratitude for others?

- How can we value the unique and individual differences among people?

- What did you like about the activities?

- What was challenging about the activities?

- What did you learn from reading *Stand Tall, Molly Lou Melon* and participating in the activities?

Thumbprint Thank-You Note Handout

These thumbprints are a unique part of me

You have always encouraged me and been able to see the real me
and helped me to be the best I can be
Thank you for all your support and all that you do
I am very grateful for you

Personal note: . . . .

. . . .

From: . . . .

Weaknesses to Strengths Handout

Weaknesses →	Strengths

THE LITTLE ENGINE THAT COULD BY WATTY PIPER

Synopsis

When their engine breaks down, the toys need another engine to pull their train over the mountain to the good little boys and girls on the other side. After several capable engines refuse to help, the toys begin to get discouraged. When a little blue engine comes along, she agrees to try to help. With the help of some positive thinking, she is able to pull the red train filled with toys and good food for the children to the other side of the mountain.

Purpose of the activity

- To promote positive thinking skills
- To encourage self-awareness and positive self-concept
- To develop coping skills

Materials needed

- Copy of *The Little Engine That Could*
- Construction paper (assorted colors)
- Scissors
- Glue
- Hole puncher
- Yarn
- Markers
- Soda in cans
- Cups
- Tacky glue

Description of the activity

Read *The Little Engine That Could* with the participants. Discuss some of the themes of the book with the group members, such as not giving up (perseverance), believing in self, using positive self-talk, and helping others. Discuss how the little train did not give up hope of finding an engine to pull them to the other side of the mountain after many of the strong and capable engines refused. Discuss how the little engine agreed to try to pull the train even though she was small and it seemed beyond her ability. Talk with the group members about the positive self-talk that the little engine used as she pulled the train to the other side of the mountain.

Activity 1: I Think I Can Train

Provide the group members with assorted colors of construction paper, scissors, glue, and markers. Ask the group members to cut a large rectangle out of one of the pieces of construction paper and two smaller circles out of a different color of the construction paper. The rectangle will serve as the train car and the small circles will serve as the wheels. If the group is short on time, these shapes can be cut out in advance. One blue engine will also need to be created from the construction paper by cutting out a blue rectangle for the body of the train, small black circles for the wheels, and a small rectangle to serve as the steam pipe for the engine.

The group members will glue their wheels to the bottom of their train car. Next, they will write an "I Can" statement on their train car using the markers. Examples might be "I can make good grades," "I can be kind to others," or "I can run a mile." These statements will be individual to each group member based on their needs and areas of focus. After the group members have written their "I Can" statements on their train cars, they can decorate them as desired using the markers. When the group have completed their train cars, the group leader can punch a hole in either end of each train car and connect them all with yarn. A hole should be punched in the back of the blue engine and it can be attached with yarn to the first train car. This makes a great bulletin board display with the heading "I Think I Can Train."

Activity 2: I Cans

(Adapted from an activity first presented by Dr. Joe Underwood and Nancy Underwood at the 2007 MCA Conference, used with prior permission.)

Explain to the group members that the group is going to have an "I Can" party to celebrate all the positive things the group members can do by drinking sodas. First, the group members have to drink sodas. If time is limited, ask them to pour their soda into cups so that the soda cans may be used more quickly. Rinse out the soda cans. Assist each group member in cutting a strip of construction paper to the size of the soda can so that it will wrap completely around it. Next, ask the group members to use the markers to draw pictures and write "I Can" statements about themselves. These statements and images should focus on goals or areas in which the group members are working to improve. Examples might be "I can manage my anger," "I can speak kind words," and "I can exercise every day." When the group members complete their "I Can" strips, assist them in gluing these around the soda cans using the tacky glue to create "I Cans" from the soda cans. If desired, all of the "I Cans" can be connected together and hung in the group area by threading yarn through the tabs on the top of the cans. This activity is also good for an individual session.

Variation of the activity

- The "I Can" statements that the group members create during the activity could also be written on small cards to keep in their pockets, binders, backpacks, handbags, etc. for frequent viewing and as a reminder to use positive self-talk daily.

Discussion questions

- Please summarize the book (*The Little Engine That Could*) we just read.

- What was your favorite part of the book?

- What was your least favorite part of the book?

- What were some of the positive traits that the little blue engine exhibited in the book?

- How did the little blue engine use positive self-talk and positive statements to help her believe in herself and pull the train over the mountain?

- Did the little blue engine believe that she could pull the train over the mountain? Explain your answer.

- What might have happened if the little blue engine was thinking or talking negatively ("I'm too small" or "I can't do it") instead of using positive self-talk and statements?

- How did the little blue engine display kindness to the train and the boys and girls on the other side of the mountain?

- Why would none of the other engines that came by pull the train over the mountain? What were some of the excuses and reasons they gave for not helping the train?

- How did all of the toys remain hopeful as they searched for an engine to help pull them to the other side of the mountain?

- What are some ways that you can use positive self-talk and positive statements in your life to help you believe in yourself?

- What is one "I Can" statement that you can use daily to encourage yourself?

- Where are some places that you can write your "I Can" statement so that you will see it frequently and remember to say it to yourself often, just as the little blue engine did in the book?

- What are some of the positive coping strategies that the train and the little blue engine used when confronted with disappointment and challenges in the book?

- What are some ways that you can help others just as the little blue engine helped the train?

- What did you like about the I Can activity?

- What was challenging about the I Can activity?

- What did you learn from reading the book and completing the I Can activity?

OH, THE PLACES YOU'LL GO BY DR. SEUSS

Synopsis

In the beginning of the book, a boy (referred to as "you") sets off a great journey with excitement and hope. As the journey unfolds, he encounters challenges and unexpected difficulties along the way. The boy copes with feelings of loneliness, fear, excitement, disappointment, and many other emotions while on his journey. Throughout the book, the boy is reminded that challenges can be overcome with hard work and positive thinking. The book also explores the themes of choices, decision making, and bad things happening to "good people."

Purpose of the activity

- To discuss and understand the importance of coping skills
- To improve self-awareness and develop positive self-concept
- To identify goals for the future and the importance of choices

Materials needed

- Copy of *Oh, The Places You'll Go*
- Assorted colors of construction paper
- Scissors
- Yarn
- Hole puncher
- Markers
- Copies of the Balloon Handout
- Collage materials (magazines and other sources of pictures and images)
- Glue

Description of the activity

Read *Oh, The Places You'll Go*. Discuss some of the themes from the book such as setting out on a journey, making choices, coping with difficulties and challenges, and the importance of hard work and believing in yourself. Discuss some of the feelings that the boy experienced on his journey and how he dealt with these. Discuss how the boy experienced difficulties and challenges even though he didn't do anything to deserve it. Discuss how the boy continued on his journey even after he dealt with challenges, difficulties, loneliness, and fear.

ACTIVITY 1: HOT AIR BALLOONS OF HOPE

In advance of the activity, cut circles (to serve as the top of the hot air balloon), squares (to serve as the base of the hot air balloon), and smaller squares (to create a design on the hot air balloon circle) from the assorted colors of construction paper. Punch holes in the sides of each circle and square and connect with a piece of the yarn to create the shape of a hot air balloon. Provide the group with the materials. On one side of the hot air balloon, ask the participants to write a coping skill or statement that will help them to maintain hope in the face of challenges. Examples might be "Stay focused on my goal," "Look for the positives," "Take time for self-care," etc. On the other side of the hot air balloon, the participants can create a mosaic or design by gluing the smaller squares of construction paper onto the larger hot air balloon circle. Discuss the coping skills or positive statements that the participants listed as well as other coping strategies to use when facing challenges.

ACTIVITY 2: THE PLACES YOU'LL GO COLLAGE

Provide the group with copies of the Balloon Handout, collage materials, scissors, and glue. Ask the group members to find pictures or words in the magazines to represent the places that they want to go during their life journey as well as any pictures or words that represent coping skills that they will need on their life journey. Ask them to cut these pictures out and glue them onto the hot air balloon shape on the handout. When complete, the hot air balloon collages can be cut out and glued to a piece of construction paper. Discuss the images that the participants selected and steps that they will need to take on their journey to make the pictures a reality. Discuss the coping skills that will be needed on the journey and how to use coping skills in various situations.

Variations of the activity

- Both of these activities work well for group or individual sessions.
- The Places You'll Go Collages make great displays for group areas or bulletin boards with the title "We're Off to Great Places."
- For long-running groups where participants may "graduate" or leave the group for various reasons, a copy of *Oh, The Places You'll Go* could be given as a gift to remind the group member of all the things he or she has learned in the group. Other group members and the group leader could write messages of support and positive statements on the front cover for the departing group member to read as a source of encouragement.

Discussion questions

- Please summarize the book (*Oh, The Places You'll Go*) that we just read.
- What was your favorite part of the book?
- What was your least favorite part of the book?
- What were some of the feelings the boy experienced throughout his journey?
- What were some of the difficulties and challenges the boy experienced on his journey?

- What were some of the skills that the boy used to cope with the challenges and difficulties?

- Did the boy do anything to deserve the challenges and difficulties that he encountered on his journey? Please explain your answer.

- How was the boy encouraged to use positive thinking while on his journey?

- How does the book end?

- What are some coping skills that you will need to use on your journey through life?

- How can you use positive thinking to help you on your journey through life?

- Tell me about the coping skills or positive statement that you wrote on your hot air balloon.

- Tell me about the images and words that you included on your collage.

- What steps will you need to take to make the images and words that you included on your collage a reality in your life?

- What did you like about the activities?

- What was challenging about the activities?

- What did you learn from the activities?

Balloon Handout

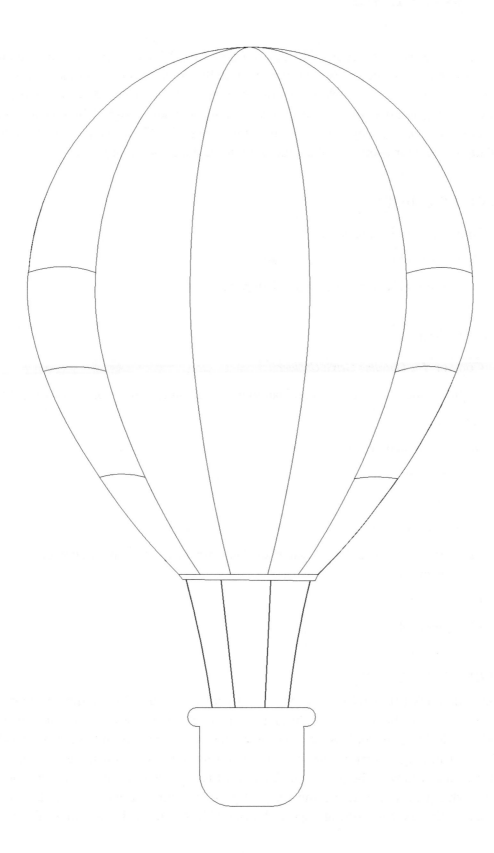

THE DUCKLING GETS A COOKIE?! BY MO WILLEMS

Synopsis

The duckling receives a cookie just by asking politely. When the pigeon comes along, he begins to complain and throw a tantrum because he did not receive a cookie. As the pigeon complains and yells, the duckling continues to remind the pigeon that he asked politely. The duckling surprises the pigeon by giving him the whole cookie. The pigeon expresses gratitude to the duckling for giving him the cookie. The book ends with the duckling asking politely for another cookie (without nuts as the duckling prefers).

Purpose of the activity

- To develop positive social skills
- To understand the importance of manners
- To develop self-control and anger management

Materials needed

- Copy of *The Duckling Gets a Cookie?!*
- Copies of the Manners are Sweet Handout (copied on card stock or heavy-weight paper)
- Scissors
- Markers, colored pencils
- Hole puncher
- Yarn, twine, ribbon
- Hand sanitizer
- Assorted variety of cookies (sugar, chocolate chip, oatmeal, peanut butter, etc.)—two per group member
- Plates, napkins, cups
- Milk (optional)

Description of the activity

Read the book (*The Duckling Gets a Cookie?!*) with the group. Discuss the behavior of the pigeon versus the behavior of the duckling in the book. What positive or negative behaviors did the duckling exhibit? What positive or negative behaviors did the pigeon exhibit? Consider making a chart on the dry erase board (if available) to list these for comparison. Discuss manners with the group members. Ask them to identify some of the manners that the duckling exhibited during the story. Did the duckling receive a cookie by using his manners? Discuss ways to use manners and social skills at school, at home, and in other settings.

Activity 1: Manners Are Sweet Booklet

Provide the participants with copies of the Manners are Sweet Handout, scissors, markers or colored pencils. Ask them to cut out each of the cookies on the Manners are Sweet Handout. On the back of each of the cookie templates, ask the participants to write one of the positive manners or social skills that was discussed after reading the book. Examples might include "Say please," "Say thank you," "Wait your turn," "Share with others." Next, ask the group members to color the front of the cookies as desired using the markers or colored pencils. When this is complete, punch holes in the side of each cookie template and tie together with yarn to create a Manners Are Sweet Booklet. The participants can use the Manners Are Sweet Booklet as a reminder to use positive manners and social skills when interacting with others.

Activity 2: Cookie Exchange Party

Explain to the group that they are going to have a Cookie Exchange Party to practice using their manners and positive social skills. Begin by having all the group members sanitize their hands. Distribute plates, cups, and milk to each of the group members. Next, give each group member a cookie (assorted variety) by placing it on their plate, but instruct them not to eat the cookie and to pick it up using the napkin provided. Explain that everyone will practice positive manners to "exchange" cookies with another group member. Everyone who participates and uses positive manners will get a surprise when the activity is complete. Begin by modeling the manners that you want the group members to exhibit by going to one of the group members and saying, "May I please exchange cookies with you?" After the group member responds, "Yes, I would like to exchange cookies," then say, "Thank you very much." Explain to the group that these are the manners and behaviors that you will be watching for as they complete the activity. Allow two group members at a time to get up and exchange cookies with other group members using the good manners modeled until all the group members have had a chance to exchange cookies. When the cookie exchange is complete, tell the group members that as their surprise for using good manners and participating in the activity, each group member can select another cookie of the variety of their choice. You may want to send home a note in advance to get permission to complete the activity and determine if any of the group members have any food allergies.

Variations of the activity

- Instead of creating a booklet with the cookie templates, each group member could write a way to exhibit good manners on the front of one of the cookie templates and color this in. A bulletin board or group display could be created with all of the cookie templates with the title "We're Smart Cookies Because We Use Good Manners!"

Discussion questions

- Please tell me about the book (*The Duckling Gets a Cookie?!*) that we just read.
- What was your favorite part of the book?
- What was your least favorite part of the book?
- How did the duckling get a cookie?
- What were some of the positive manners and social skills that the duckling used in the book?
- How did the pigeon behave when he arrived and realized that the duckling had a cookie?
- What were some of the negative behaviors that the pigeon exhibited when he did not have a cookie?
- How did the duckling tell the pigeon that he asked for a cookie?
- What did the duckling do with his cookie?
- How did the pigeon respond when the duckling gave him his cookie? What manners did the pigeon use when he was given the cookie?
- What positive manners did the duckling use to receive another cookie?
- What are some manners and social skills that you use to get along with others?
- What did you like about the activities?
- What was challenging about the activities?
- What did you learn from participating in the activities?

Manners are Sweet Handout

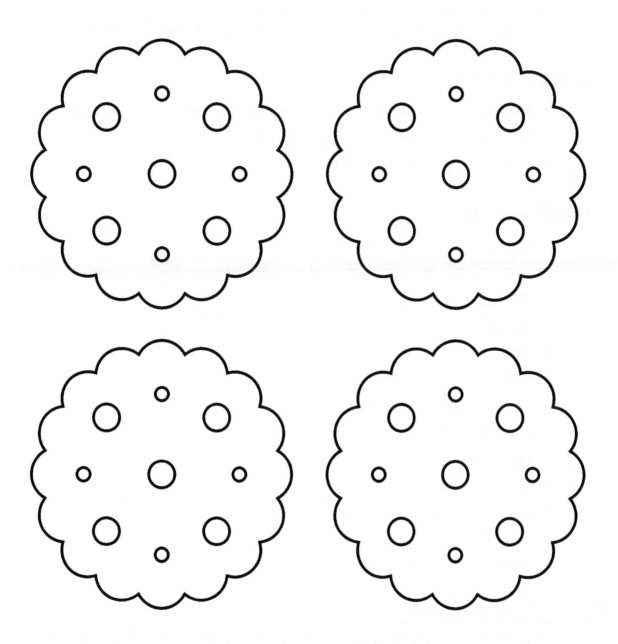

THE VERY HUNGRY CATERPILLAR BY ERIC CARLE

Synopsis

The book begins with a tiny caterpillar hatching from an egg. He is hungry and begins to eat through several different types of fruit for five days, but on the sixth day, the hungry caterpillar eats a variety of junk food and experiences a stomach ache. After eating a green leaf, the caterpillar feels better. He then creates himself a cocoon. He stays in the cocoon for two weeks, pushes himself out of the cocoon, and becomes a beautiful butterfly.

Purpose of the activity

- To develop self-awareness and an understanding of the importance of self-care
- To identify self-care strategies and coping skills
- To encourage persistence toward goals

Materials needed

- Copy of *The Very Hungry Caterpillar*
- Oranges, apples, strawberries, pears, plums (cut these into pieces in advance)
- Plates
- Napkins
- Forks
- Copies of the Healthy Caterpillar Handout
- Markers, crayons, colored pencils
- Clothespin
- Pipe cleaners
- Tissue paper
- Scissors
- Tacky glue
- Magnets with adhesive back

Description of the activity

Read *The Very Hungry Caterpillar* with the group. Discuss the food choices that the caterpillar made. Discuss how the caterpillar felt after eating the healthy fruit compared with how he felt after eating lots of junk food. Discuss some of the reasons that the caterpillar had to build a cocoon, such as the need to rest and grow to become a butterfly. Discuss what might have happened if the caterpillar did not push himself out and instead chose to remain in the cocoon. Discuss the importance of making healthy choices and having persistence toward goals in our lives.

ACTIVITY 1: HEALTHY CATERPILLAR, HEALTHY ME

Begin by telling the group members that they are going to have a fruit tasting today. Many healthy foods such as fruit taste good and are good for our bodies. It is important to make good choices about our physical and mental health. Provide each group member with a plate, napkin, fork, and a sample of each of the fruits. As the group members are eating, discuss specific changes and steps that each group member can take to become more physically and mentally healthy. When the group members have finished eating, distribute copies of the Healthy Caterpillar Handout as well as the writing supplies. Ask the participants to write one way to stay healthy either physically or mentally in each of the sections of the caterpillar. When finished, they can color or decorate their caterpillars. Discuss the strategies to stay healthy that the group members listed on their caterpillars and ways that they can implement these strategies in their lives.

ACTIVITY 2: BUTTERFLY REMINDER

Butterflies are beautiful creatures that are often associated with life, freedom, and positive change. Every butterfly first starts as a caterpillar and must persevere through challenges, waiting periods, and hard work to become a butterfly. Just as the caterpillar in the book had to eat healthy foods, build a cocoon, rest and wait in the cocoon, and then push himself out to become a butterfly, we have to persevere through trials, waiting periods, and challenges in order to reach our goals. Explain to the group members that they are going to create a butterfly magnet to serve as a reminder for them to persevere through challenges and to keep working toward their goals so that they can become "butterflies." Provide the group members with the clothespin (body of caterpillar), pipe cleaners (cut to be the butterfly's antennae), tissue paper (cut to be the butterfly's wings), scissors, tacky glue, and magnetic strip. Assist them in gluing the pipe cleaner pieces to the top of the clothespin to serve as the butterfly's antennae. Glue the two tissue paper wings to the inside of the clothespin. Pull the adhesive backing off of the magnetic strip and attach to the back of the clothespin. If desired, the group members can color the clothespin with markers or draw a face on it. Discuss with the group members ways that the butterfly can serve as a reminder to them to persevere to reach their goals.

Discussion questions

- Please summarize the book (*The Very Hungry Caterpillar*) we just read.
- What was your favorite part of the book?
- What was your least favorite part of the book?
- How did the caterpillar feel after eating the healthy fruit in the book?
- How did the caterpillar feel after overeating on all the junk food?
- What happened while the caterpillar was in the cocoon?
- What did the caterpillar have to do to get out of the cocoon?
- Why is it important to take care of our physical and mental health?
- What are some ways to stay physically healthy?
- What are some ways to stay mentally healthy?

- What are some of the ways that the caterpillar showed perseverance in order to become a butterfly?

- What is an area in your life in which you need to show perseverance in order to achieve a goal?

- What are some of the positive things that a butterfly symbolizes?

- Where will you put your Butterfly Reminder so that you remember to persevere and work hard toward becoming a "butterfly?"

- What did you like about the activities?

- What was challenging about the activities?

- What did you learn from completing the activities?

Healthy Caterpillar Handout

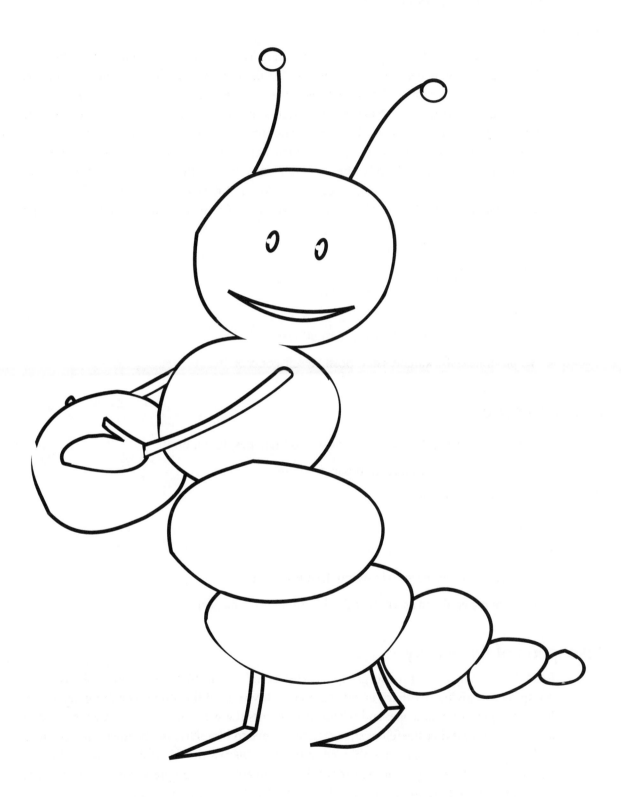

THE GIVING TREE
BY SHEL SILVERSTEIN

Synopsis

The book begins with a boy and an apple tree. The boy enjoys playing with the tree, swinging on the branches and eating the fruit. As the boy grows older, his interests change. First, the boy wants money. The tree suggests he sells her apples to make money. The tree is happy to give to the boy. Next, the boy wants to build a house. The tree offers for the boy to cut her branches to build his house. The tree is happy to give to the boy. Later, the boy wants a boat. The tree suggests that he cut her trunk to make a boat so the boy cuts her trunk to make a boat. Finally, the boy (an elderly man at this point in the story) comes to the tree again. The tree feels sad because she does not have anything left to give, but the boy only wants a place to rest which he finds by sitting on the tree stump. The tree is happy to give to the boy.

Purpose of the activity

- To develop positive social skills
- To identify and learn ways to give to others
- To promote self-awareness and positive self-concept

Materials needed

- Large piece of paper with a tree trunk and branches drawn on it
- Assorted colors of construction paper
- Markers, pencils, pens
- Scissors
- Glue
- Copies of the My Personal Giving Tree Handout
- Collage materials (magazines and other sources of images)

Description of the activity

Read *The Giving Tree* with the group. Discuss some of the themes of the book with the group such as giving to others, unconditional positive regard for others, changing needs and interests as we grow and age, and friendship. Discuss the ways that the tree gave to the boy and the happiness that she felt as she was able to give to him. Discuss the unconditional love and positive regard that the tree showed to the boy. Discuss the friendship between the boy and the tree and the ways that their friendship changed as the boy grew. Discuss the concept of giving with the group members and how they feel about giving to others.

Activity 1: Giving Handprint Tree

Begin by distributing the construction paper, scissors, and writing supplies to the group members. Explain that they are going to create a Giving Handprint Tree. Ask the group members to trace their hand on the construction paper and cut it out using the scissors. Next, ask them to write a way that they can give to others on the handprint. They can also decorate their handprints. Once this is complete, assist all of the group members in gluing their handprints to the branches of the tree drawn on the large piece of paper. Ask them to share the ways that they identified to give to others as they attach their handprints to the Giving Handprint Tree. The Giving Handprint Tree makes a great display for bulletin boards or group spaces.

Activity 2: My Personal Giving Tree Collage

Explain to the group that they are going to create a collage of ways to give to others. Provide them with the My Personal Giving Tree Handout and other needed supplies. Ask the group members to cut images, words, and phrases from the magazines and other image sources that depict ways to give to others. Next, ask them to glue these images to the handout. When this has been completed, ask the participants to share their giving tree collages with the group and talk about the images, words, and phrases that they have selected.

Variations of the activity

- If there is not enough time in the group to complete the Giving Handprint Tree, the My Personal Giving Tree Handout could be used to create a thumbprint tree. Cut out the tree template and glue to a piece of construction paper. Ask each group member to press their thumbprint in an ink pad and press to make a thumbprint on the tree. Using a pen, each group member can write a way to give back to others next to their thumbprint.

- The Giving Handprint Tree activity also works well for an activity for family therapy.

Discussion questions

- Please summarize the book (*The Giving Tree)* that we just read.

- What was your favorite part of the book?

- What was your least favorite part of the book?

- What were some of the ways that the tree gave to the boy?

- How did the tree feel after she gave to the boy?

- How did the tree show unconditional love and positive regard to the boy?

- How did the boy's friendship with the tree change as he grew up?

- What did the boy give to the tree?

- Did the tree receive anything in return for all that she gave to the boy? Explain your answer.

- Is it better to give or to receive? Explain your answer.

- Why is it important to give to others?
- What are a few ways that you can give back to others without expecting anything in return?
- What did you like about the activities?
- What was challenging about the activities?
- What did you learn from participating in the activities and reading *The Giving Tree?*

My Personal Giving Tree Handout

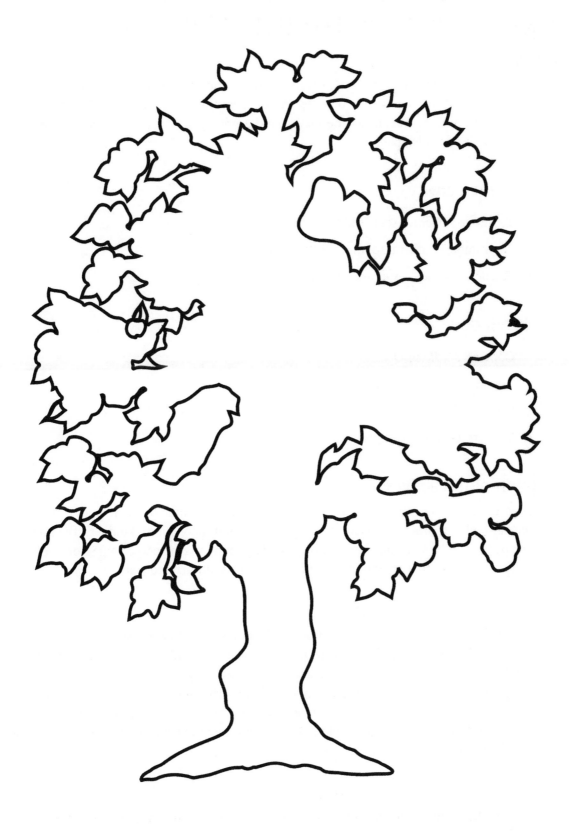

THE RECESS QUEEN
BY ALEXIS O'NEILL (AUTHOR) AND
LAURA HULISKA-BEITH (ILLUSTRATOR)

Synopsis

Mean Jean rules the playground at her school. She bullies the other children, and they are all afraid of her. When a new girl comes to school, everything changes. Katie Sue is not afraid of Mean Jean. Katie Sue makes the playground a great place again by teaching Jean about kindness and friendship.

Purpose of the activity

- To develop positive social skills

- To promote conflict resolution skills

- To encourage self-awareness and positive self-concept

Materials needed

- Copy of *The Recess Queen*

- Copies of the Ideal Playground Handouts

- Large piece of paper

- Markers, pens, colored pencils

Description of the activity

Read the book (*The Recess Queen*) with the group. Discuss some of the themes of the book such as bullying (from the perspective of the bully and the victims), kindness, the power of one person, and friendship. Discuss how the playground was able to change from a place of bullying and fear to a great place through Katie Sue's kindness to Jean.

ACTIVITY 1: IDEAL PLAYGROUND—INDIVIDUAL

Distribute copies of the Ideal Playground Handouts and drawing supplies to the group members. Explain that they are each going to create their ideal playground. On the first handout, ask the group members to draw their ideal playground. The only limit is their imagination. They can include slides, swings, bounce houses, etc. On the second handout, ask them to identify positive ways to interact with others in the playground and to create a Playground Bill of Rights that would help the playground remain a positive place to interact socially with others.

ACTIVITY 2: IDEAL PLAYGROUND—GROUP MURAL

Provide the group members with a large sheet of paper and drawing supplies. Ask them to work together to create an Ideal Playground and A Playground Bill of Rights on the mural paper. If the group members have already completed Activity 1, then they can each bring their individual Ideal Playground and Playground Bill of Rights Handouts to discuss as they create the group mural. When the Ideal Playground mural and the Playground Bill of Rights are complete, ask the group members to talk about them and how they were developed.

Variations of the activity

- If possible, allow the group members to play on a nearby playground or take a trip to a local park so that they can practice using some of the positive social skills that they have learned about in the book and through completing the activities.

Discussion questions

- Please summarize the book (*The Recess Queen*) that we just read.
- What was your favorite part of the book?
- What was your least favorite part of the book?
- Describe Mean Jean.
- How did the other children feel about Mean Jean?
- What did Mean Jean do on the playground?
- Did Mean Jean have many friends? Explain your answer.
- Describe Katie Sue.
- How did Katie Sue respond when Mean Jean tried to bully her on the playground?
- What did Katie Sue ask Jean to do that no one had ever asked her to do before?
- How did Jean become Katie Sue's friend?
- How did Katie Sue make the playground a better place for everyone just by being kind to Jean?
- Has someone ever bullied you or acted like Mean Jean did at the beginning of the book? How did you handle it?
- How can you be kind to others even if they are not kind to you?
- Tell me about your Ideal Playground.
- Tell me about your Playground Bill of Rights.
- What are some ways to interact positively with others?
- How would you handle it if you saw someone else being bullied?
- What can you do to spread kindness in the places you go?
- What did you like about the activities?
- What was challenging about the activities?
- What did you learn from the activities?

Ideal Playground Handout

Use the space below to create your ideal playground:

Ideal Playground Bill of Rights Handout

Use the space below to create an Ideal Playground Bill of Rights to keep the playground a safe and happy place for all children:

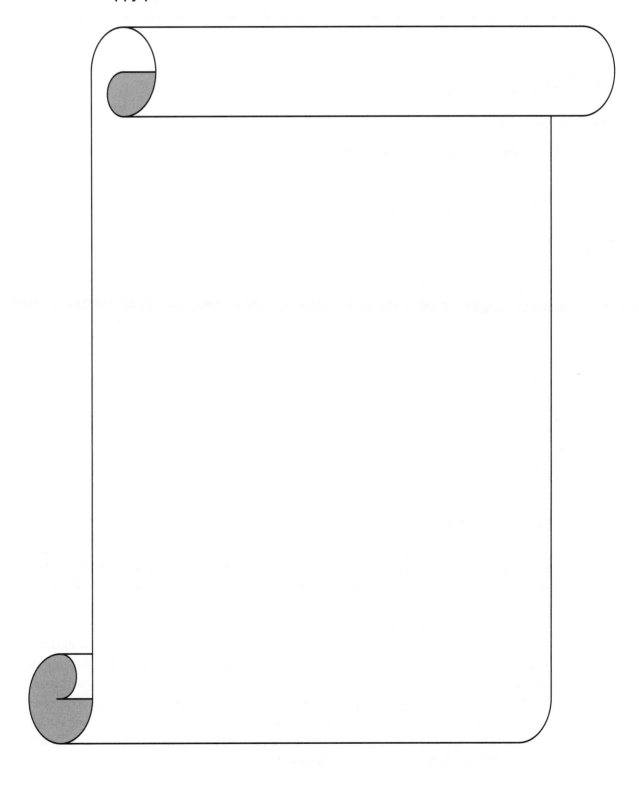

CHAPTER 6

Hands-On Activities

EGGING IT ON

Purpose of the activity

- To understand the power of words and actions
- To develop self-awareness
- To promote conflict resolution skills

Materials needed

- Empty egg shells (intact to hold paint)
- Egg carton
- Tissue paper
- Scissors
- Tape or glue
- Art canvas
- Drop cloth
- Assorted colors of paint

Description of the activity

In advance of the session, fill the empty egg shells with paint (one color per egg). Cut a small piece of tissue paper and glue or tape over the opening of the egg. Place each paint-filled egg in the egg carton. Cover the area where painting will occur with a drop cloth. Place the art canvas on top of the drop cloth.

When the participant arrives, begin by asking if she has ever said or done anything that she wished she hadn't or if someone has ever said or done something to her that hurt her feelings or was hard for her to forget about after it happened. Explain that she is going to participate in an activity to illustrate the power of words and actions. Provide the participant with the carton of paint-filled eggs. Ask her to throw the eggs on the art canvas. The paint-filled eggs will make splatter marks and designs all over the art canvas, creating a piece of abstract art. After the participant has thrown all of the eggs, allow the art canvas to dry and discuss the activity with her using the discussion questions.

Variations of the activity

- Egging It On also works well as a group activity.

- Consider using different types of materials instead of the art canvas. Options to consider include white t-shirts, canvas bags, poster-board, mural paper.

Discussion questions

- Tell me about a time when you said something or did something that you later wished you hadn't said or done.

- Tell me about a time when someone else said or did something that hurt or upset you and that you had difficulty forgetting about afterwards.

- Why are words and actions powerful?

- How can our words and actions be used in a positive way?

- How can our words and actions be used in a harmful way?

- How long did it take to throw the paint-filled eggs on the canvas?

- How long will the paint remain on the canvas once it has been thrown?

- How does this activity represent the lasting impact of our words and actions? (It only took a short time to throw the paint-filled eggs, but the paint will remain on the canvas for a long time. Similarly, it only takes moment to say or do something in anger, but the impact of those words or actions can last a very long time.)

- If our words and actions are so powerful, why do we use them in hurtful ways at times?

- What are some ways that we can resolve conflicts without saying or doing things that we will later regret?

- How can you handle it if you do say or do something that you wish you hadn't done? What are some steps that you can take to resolve the situation?

- How can you handle it if someone does or says something that hurts you? What are some ways to let go of things that have hurt or upset you in the past?

- How can you focus on being mindful of the words that you say and the things that you do in the future?

- What did you like about this activity?

- What was challenging about this activity?

- What did you learn from participating in this activity?

BROKEN BEAUTY

Purpose of the activity

- To develop positive thinking skills
- To promote self-awareness and positive self-concept
- To encourage coping skills

Materials needed

- Sidewalk chalk (assorted colors)
- Ziploc bags
- Hammer or rolling pin
- Small bowls
- Water
- Paint brushes
- Art paper

Description of the activity

As the participant watches, place the sidewalk chalk in a Ziploc bags (one color per bag), seal, and crush into a fine powder with either the hammer or the rolling pin. Discuss with the participant how the sidewalk chalk is now broken. Discuss if the broken pieces are now useless and should just be thrown away. Next, pour the chalk powder into the small bowls and slowly add water to create a paint-like consistency. Ask the participant if the powder has now become useful again. Explain that the crushed powder that appeared broken can now be used to paint a beautiful picture. Provide the participant with art paper and brushes in order to paint with the repurposed chalk paint. As the participant paints, discuss how the example of the broken beauty of the chalk paint can also apply to our lives. Many times we may make a mistake or do something we regret and feel that we are now "useless," but we can always become something new and beautiful even if we have become "broken" in some way.

Variations of the activity

- Depending on the age of the participant, you could allow her to crush the sidewalk chalk with the rolling pin.
- Glitter can be added to the chalk powder for a fun effect. The glitter can represent the support and encouragement we receive from others when we feel "down" or "broken."

Discussion questions

- (After putting sidewalk chalk in Ziploc bags.) What do you see?

- (After crushing sidewalk chalk.) What has happened to the sidewalk chalk now?

- Is this sidewalk chalk broken and useless now?

- Should we just throw the broken chalk powder away?

- (After adding water and creating chalk paint.) What has happened to the broken chalk powder now?

- How did the broken chalk powder that seemed useless become useful again?

- What can you now create with the chalk paint?

- How can the broken chalk paint example be applied to our lives?

- Have you ever felt "broken," "useless," or as if you have made too many mistakes? Explain your answer.

- How can the example of the chalk paint becoming useful and beautiful again when it seemed broken and useless apply to our lives?

- Can you think of a time when you were able to use something that made you feel broken in a positive way or to help others?

- What are some ways that we can learn from mistakes and past experiences and use them in positive ways in the future?

- What are some positive ways to cope with making mistakes or feeling useless?

- Where will you display your Broken Beauty chalk painting to be reminded that even things that are seemingly broken can be changed into something beautiful and positive?

- What did you like about this activity?

- What was challenging about this activity?

- What did you learn from participating in this activity?

COLOR ME _____

Purpose of the activity

- To identify feelings and emotions and ways that feelings and emotions impact us
- To promote self-awareness
- To identify positive ways to cope with feelings and emotions

Materials needed

- Clear plastic cups
- Sprite
- Ice cube tray
- Access to a freezer
- Powdered Kool-Aid (red and blue)
- Water

Description of the activity

In advance of the session, pour red powdered Kool-Aid in some of the openings of the ice cube tray and blue powered Kool-Aid in the remaining openings of the ice cube tray. Then pour water into the openings on top of the powered Kool-Aid and place in the freezer for at least three to four hours. When it is time for the session, pour Sprite into three of the clear plastic cups. Ask the participant to think about an emotion that is commonly associated with the color red. Red is often associated with anger (e.g. I'm so mad that I'm seeing red). Ask the participant to pretend that the red Kool-Aid ice cubes represent anger. Ask her to think of an emotion that is associated with the color blue. Blue is often associated with feeling sad (e.g. I've really been feeling blue about my friend moving away). Ask the participant to pretend that the blue ice cubes represent sadness. Place the cups of Sprite on the table. Place the red ice cubes in one of the cups of Sprite, the blue ice cubes in the second cup of Sprite, and leave the third cup just plain Sprite. Ask the participant to imagine that the clear Sprite represents someone who is coping with all of their emotions in a healthy and balanced way at the present time. The cup with red ice cubes represents someone who is struggling with anger and anger management, and the cup with blue ice cubes represents someone who is struggling with sadness and depression. As the ice cubes melt, the Sprite will change to red in the anger cup and blue in the sadness cup. Discuss the activity with the participant using the discussion questions below.

Variations of the activity

- The Sprite with Kool-Aid ice cubes could be used as a fun drink for the participant after the activity.
- This activity also works well for group sessions.

Discussion questions

- What is an emotion associated with the color red?

- What does the expression "I'm seeing red" mean?

- What is an emotion associated with the color blue?

- What does the expression "I'm feeling blue" mean?

- What does it feel like when you are emotionally healthy and balanced?

- Have you ever felt as if an emotion like anger or sadness was "taking over" your life? Describe this time in your life.

- What happens when we do not deal with our emotions and feelings or express them in a healthy way?

- What happens to the Sprite when we add the red "anger" ice cubes to one cup and the blue "sadness" ice cubes to the other cup? (The red "anger" color takes over its cup and the blue "sadness" color takes over its cup.)

- How is the Sprite and Kool-Aid ice cubes activity an example of the way our emotions take over when we don't deal with them in a healthy manner?

- What are some unhealthy ways that people deal with emotions such as anger and sadness?

- What are some healthy ways to cope with emotions such as anger and sadness?

- What is one new strategy that you can use to cope with your emotions in a positive manner?

- What did you like about this activity?

- What was challenging about this activity?

- What did you learn from completing this activity?

STOMP ROCKET DE-ESCALATION

Purpose of the activity

- To identify ways to de-escalate situations
- To learn ways to manage anger
- To promote conflict resolution skills

Materials needed

- Stomp rocket
- Outdoor space to complete the activity

Description of the activity

Begin by setting up the stomp rocket in an open space outdoors. Explain to the participant that the discussion today will be about de-escalation and the stomp rocket will be used to facilitate the discussion. Allow the participant to jump on the launch pad and make the stomp rocket shoot up several times. After she has done this a few times, ask her to jump as hard as she can on the launch pad and note how high the stomp rocket goes in the air. Next, ask her to jump very lightly on the launch pad and discuss how high the rocket goes in the air. The harder the participant jumps on the launch pad, the higher the rocket will shoot into the sky. Discuss with the participant how this relates to de-escalation. If someone is upset and we "jump" on them by yelling back or making unkind remarks, then the person may become more upset and the situation is likely to escalate. However, if someone is upset and we just handle it very lightly by using a calm approach and kind words, the situation is likely to de-escalate. It is the same principle as with the stomp rocket. When we only press lightly on the launch pad, it will not go very high (or escalate), but when we put lots of pressure by jumping hard on the launch pad, it will shoot high in the sky (or escalate). Allow the participant to continue playing with the stomp rocket if time allows. Conclude by discussing other ways to manage anger, and resolve conflicts to ensure that the situation is de-escalated.

Variations of the activity

- This activity also works well with groups.

Discussion questions

- What does the word de-escalation mean?
- What does it mean to escalate a situation?
- Please give an example of how the situation might escalate to an angry outburst when a person is upset.
- Please give an example of how the situation might de-escalate when a person who is upset becomes calm again.

- Describe how the stomp rocket works.

- What happens if you jump very hard on the launch pad? How high does the rocket shoot?

- What happens if you only press lightly on the launch pad? How does the rocket shoot?

- How does the stomp rocket example relate to the process of de-escalation?

- What are some ways that a person might escalate a situation by "jumping hard?"

- What are some ways that a person could de-escalate a situation by "stepping lightly?"

- How can the principle of the way the stomp rocket works guide you in resolving conflicts with others?

- How can you change the way you approach a person who is angry or upset in order to de-escalate the situation instead of escalate it?

- What did you like about this activity?

- What was challenging about this activity?

- What did you learn from completing this activity?

RAINBOW POTS

Purpose of the activity

- To appreciate diversity and difference among individuals

- To promote self-awareness and positive self-concept

- To develop positive thinking skills

Materials needed

- Terracotta pot (one per participant)

- Assorted colors of acrylic paint (in tubes or bottles)

- Drop cloth to cover area

- Smocks or old t-shirts to protect clothing

Description of the activity

In advance of the activity, prepare the area where painting will take place by putting a drop cloth over the ground (acrylic paint will stain). Place the terracotta pot on the drop cloth with the bottom side up. When the participant arrives, ask her to put on a smock or old t-shirt to protect her clothing. Ask her what she notices about the terracotta pot. Point out that right now it is only one color and does not have much diversity. Provide the participant with the assorted colors of acrylic paint. Help her to get started by squeezing the tube or bottle of paint down the side of the pot. Rotate the pot and drizzle each color a few times down the side of the pot. Ask the participant to repeat the process with the various colors of paint. Ask her to use at least five colors of paint. Continue with the process until the whole pot is covered with assorted colors of paint drizzled down the side. Allow the pot to dry over night. After the participant has finished painting, discuss what the pot looks like now. Discuss the beauty and diversity of all the different colors on the pot. Ask how the example of the pot applies to people and diversity and difference among people. Discuss ways to appreciate diversity and difference among other people.

Variations of the activity

- This activity works well for groups.

- If desired, a plant or flower could be added to each pot. The Rainbow Pots make great gifts for the participants to give to someone.

- Consider serving a rainbow-colored snack when the activity is complete for a fun conclusion to the session.

Discussion questions

- What does the word "diversity" mean?

- What do you notice about the pot (before painting)?

- What does diversity do for our world? What would the world be like if there was no diversity and everyone was exactly the same?

- Why do you think the pots are called Rainbow Pots?

- What do you notice about the pot now that it is painted? How would you describe the pot?

- What are some types of diversity among people?

- How does diversity make the world a more beautiful and exciting place?

- What are some ways that you can appreciate diversity and difference among people?

- How can we show respect for people who are different from us?

- How can we learn from people who are different from us?

- What did you like about this activity?

- What was challenging about this activity?

- What did you learn from participating in this activity?

BLOWING AWAY OUR WORRIES

Purpose of the activity

- To develop healthy coping skills
- To encourage positive thinking skills
- To promote self-awareness

Materials needed

- Bubbles with wands (several bottles)
- Assorted colors of food coloring
- Large piece of paper
- Tape
- Outdoor wall to use to hang paper

Description of the activity

In advance of the activity, tape the paper to the wall. Mix one color of food coloring into each bottle of bubbles. When the participant arrives, discuss what it means to be worried or anxious and ask her how it feels. Sometimes, worries seem to get "stuck" in our heads and be the only thing that we can think about or focus on. Explain to the participant that today she is going to participate in an activity to "blow" her worries away. If desired, the different colors of bubbles could represent different areas of life. For example, the bubbles with red food coloring could represent relationship worries, the bubbles with blue food coloring could represent worries about school, etc. Ask the participant to stand relatively close to the paper, select the desired bottle of bubbles, and blow them at the paper. As the participant blows the bubbles, ask her to visualize that she is blowing the things she is worried about away. The paper will "catch" the bubbles (the bubbles will make an impression on the paper when they hit it). The participant can repeat this process with the different colors of bubbles and continue to visualize blowing away worries and negativity. When the activity is complete, ask the participant to visualize that all of the worries and negativity have been removed from her. Assist her in developing positive affirmations and replacement thoughts to use in place of the worries.

Variations of the activity

- This activity also works well for group sessions.
- If time allows, the participant can use markers or pens to write positive affirmations and replacement thoughts for each worry or negative thought she "blew away" on and around the bubble impressions on the piece of paper. This makes a great display with the heading "We are Letting Our Positive Thoughts Bubble Up."

Discussion questions

- What does it mean to worry or to be worried?

- What does it mean to be anxious?

- What does it feel like when you are worried or anxious?

- Do you ever get worries or negative thoughts "stuck" in your head? If so, describe how this feels.

- What are some of the things that you are worried about right now? What are some situations or events that can trigger you to worry or feel anxious?

- What did it feel like to visualize "blowing your worries" away?

- Why is it not helpful to worry or dwell on negative thoughts?

- How did it feel to see all of your worries stuck on the paper and removed from you?

- What are some positive thoughts or replacement thoughts that you can use if you begin to feel worried or have negative thoughts?

- What are some other coping strategies that you can use when you feel worried or anxious?

- What is one new strategy that you can use in your life to deal with worry, anxiety, or negative thoughts?

- What did you like about this activity?

- What was challenging about this activity?

- What did you learn from completing this activity?

RELEASING NEGATIVITY

Purpose of the activity

- To promote positive thinking
- To develop self-awareness and positive self-concept
- To encourage healthy coping skills

Materials needed

- Balloons
- Access to a helium tank
- Strings for balloons
- Small pieces of paper
- Pens
- Access to outdoor space

Description of the activity

Begin by discussing negative thoughts and worries with the participant. Discuss how hard it can be to let go of things that have hurt us, negative thought patterns, and worries. Discuss the impact of holding on to negativity and worries. Explain to the participant that the activity will be a balloon release to "let go and release" all of the negativity and worries that she has been holding onto and that may be holding her back in some way. Provide the participant with the small strips of paper. Ask her to write any negative thoughts, things that have hurt her that she is holding on to, or worries on the strips of paper. When complete, she can fold these up and place the small pieces of paper inside the balloons. Next, the balloons can be filled with helium and tied with a string. After the balloons are filled and tied, ask the participant to step outside with the balloons. Countdown with the participant and ask her to "let go and release" the balloons along with all of the negative thoughts, worries, and past hurts. Discuss ways to replace these thoughts with positive affirmations and replacement thoughts.

Variations of the activity

- This also works well as a group activity.
- Participants can make one balloon for each worry or negative thought or put all of the worries and negative thoughts in one balloon.

Discussion questions

- Have you ever had a negative thought, worry, or something that hurt you that you had trouble letting go of? Please tell me about it.

- What does it mean to "let it go?"

- How do you know if you have really "let go" of a worry, negative thought, or past hurt?

- What are the differences between "holding on to" a negative thought, worry, or past hurt and "letting go" of it?

- What are some of the things that stop of us from "letting go" of negativity?

- What are some worries, negative thoughts, or past hurts that you want to release and let go of?

- How did it feel to write all of the things on the strips and then watch them float away inside the balloon?

- What strategies can you use to make sure you don't try to take back all of the worries and negative thoughts that you released today?

- What are some positive affirmations and thoughts that you can use in place of the worries and negative thoughts you have let go of?

- What are some other healthy ways to cope when you have negative thoughts or feel worried?

- What is one new strategy you can use to deal with worries and negative thoughts?

- What did you like about this activity?

- What was challenging about this activity?

- What did you learn from completing this activity?

COVERED IN SLIME

Purpose of the activity

- To develop self-awareness and positive self-concept
- To understand the impact of our choices and decisions
- To encourage positive social skills

Materials needed

- Cornstarch
- Water
- Food coloring or paint
- Bowl
- Drop cloth

Description of the activity

Begin by discussing some of the influences in the participant's life. Discuss positive versus negative influences and the consequences of surrounding ourselves with negative influences. Explain to the participant that she is going to make slime today to illustrate some of the impacts of negative influences and making bad choices. Provide her with the needed supplies. In the bowl, add one cup of cornstarch. Next, slowly add water (approximately two cups) and food coloring or paint (if desired). Ask the participant to mix the ingredients with her hands until it reaches the consistency of a thick, slimy liquid. Discuss with the participant how surrounding ourselves with negative influences and making choices that lead down negative paths is similar to being covered in slime. Discuss with her some of the steps that she can take to remove herself from negative influences or to make positive changes in her life in response to previous negative choices. Compare the cleaning and removal of slime to the removal of negative influences in life. (Slime can be removed with warm water. Be sure to put slime in the garbage can and not down the drain as it can clog up the sink). Discuss ways to make positive changes and cope with negative influences.

Variations of the activity

- This is also a fun activity for groups.
- Consider making a "slimy" snack such as jello or pudding for a fun conclusion to the activity.

Discussion questions

- What are some of the positive influences in your life?
- What are some of the negative influences in your life?

- What are some of the consequences of surrounding yourself with negative influences?

- What are some of the benefits of surrounding yourselves with positive influences?

- How does the slime feel on your hands?

- How does the slime that we made compare to negative influences in our lives? (The slime is sticky and covers your hands. Similarly, when we get involved with bad influences, we often become "stuck" and "covered" by the negative influences.)

- What are some ways to separate yourself from negative influences?

- How can you cope with negative influences that cannot be removed from your life?

- How can you surround yourself with more positive influences?

- What are some ways to evaluate your choices and decisions to make sure that they won't lead to negative consequences?

- What are some steps you can take to make positive decisions and choices in life?

- How did you clean and remove the slime from your hands?

- How is removing negative influences from your life similar to removing and cleaning the slime from your hands?

- What did you like about this activity?

- What was challenging about this activity?

- What did you learn from completing this activity?

ERUPTING ANGER

Purpose of the activity

- To develop anger management skills
- To learn about de-escalation
- To promote self-awareness

Materials needed

- Diet Sprite (two liter)
- Mentos mints
- Red food coloring or red paint
- Large piece of paper or cardboard

Description of the activity

Begin by discussing with the participant what it feels like to be angry. Ask her if she has ever had an angry outburst or a temper tantrum. Ask the participant to describe what happened and what it felt like when the angry outburst or tantrum occurred. Often, angry outbursts are compared to an eruption or explosion. Discuss what happens during an eruption or explosion. Explain that during the activity today, she will create an actual eruption and then compare it to how an angry outburst occurs. Place the paper or cardboard on the ground. Open the two-liter bottle of Diet Sprite and add red food coloring or paint. Next, drop in the Mentos mints and wait for the eruption. This happens very quickly so be sure the participant is ready and watching. Discuss how the Diet Sprite and Mentos mint eruption compares to an angry outburst. Both happen very quickly, but then have lasting impacts. Discuss how the red paint or food coloring left spots and stains on the paper. In the same way, our angry outbursts may hurt others around us. Discuss ways to manage anger, resolve conflicts, and de-escalate situations to prevent angry outbursts.

Variations of the activity

- This activity also works well with groups.
- Consider getting several two-liter bottles of Sprite and packs of Mentos mints so that the activity can be completed a few times. It happens very quickly and it helps if the participant can observe it more than once during the session to illustrate some of the discussion points.

Discussion questions

- What does it feel like to be angry?

- Describe a time when you had an angry outburst or temper tantrum. What happened? What did it feel like? How quickly did it happen? How long did it last? What happened afterwards?

- What is an eruption? Where does an eruption occur? What are the impacts of an eruption?

- Describe what happened when we added the Mentos mints to the Diet Sprite. How quickly did the eruption occur? How long did it last? What were some of the impacts of the eruption?

- How does the Diet Sprite and Mentos mints eruption compare to an angry outburst or temper tantrum?

- What are some of the impacts or consequences of an angry outburst?

- What are some strategies that you can use to avoid angry outbursts?

- What are some ways to resolve conflicts with others without becoming angry or having an angry outburst?

- If you have already had an angry outburst, what can you do to repair the relationship or reverse some of the impacts of this?

- What are some signs that you are about to have an angry outburst?

- How can you use your anger management strategies to de-escalate the situation?

- What did you like about this activity?

- What was challenging about this activity?

- What did you learn from completing this activity?

Resources

For art and craft supplies

Art Discount: www.artdiscount.co.uk
Dick Blick Art Supplies: www.dickblick.com
Great Art: www.greatart.co.uk
Lawrence Art supplies: www.lawrence.co.uk
Oriental Trading Company: www.orientaltrading.com
S&S Worldwide: www.ssww.com

For books and games

Amazon (United States): www.amazon.com
Amazon (United Kingdom): www.amazon.co.uk
Amazon (Canada): www.amazon.ca
Barnes & Noble (United States): www.barnesandnoble.com
Books-A-Million (United States): www.booksamillion.com

For information about holidays

USA Government: www.usa.gov/citizens/holidays.shtml

Index of Purposes of Activities

Purpose	Activity	Page number
Communication skills *cont.*	Inside My Head Silhouette	95
	We All Blend Together Color Wheel	124
	Improving Our World Handprint Wreath (Dr. Martin Luther King Jr.'s Birthday)	140
	String of Hearts (Valentine's Day)	143
	Mother's Day Flower	160
	A Mother's Day Interview (Mother's Day)	163
	Nature Scavenger Hunt (Fall)	186
Anger management	What Gets Me Bent out of Shape?	63
	Paint Chip Reminder Strips	87
	Bad Hair Day Art	117
	Reminder Rings	130
	Relaxation Playdough Balloons	158
	Cooling Down My Anger Ice Cream Party (Summer)	166
	I'm Feeling Crabby (Summer)	172
	Melting Away Our Anger Mini Pumpkins (Halloween/Fall)	192
	Bibliotherapy: *The Duckling Gets a Cookie?!* (Manners are Sweet and Cookie Exchange)	220
	Stomp Rocket De-escalation	242
	Erupting Anger	252
Conflict resolution	Improving Our World Handprint Wreath (Dr. Martin Luther King Jr.'s Birthday)	140
	Bibliotherapy: *The Recess Queen* (Ideal Playground—Individual and Group)	232
	Melting Away Our Anger Mini Pumpkins (Fall)	192
	Egging It On	236
	Stomp Rocket De-escalation	242
Goal setting	Diamond in the Rough	46
	Reaching for Our Stars	55
	Putting My Best Foot Forward in the New Year	137
	Pot of Gold Goals Collage (St. Patrick's Day)	151
	Keys to Success (Preparing for going back to school)	178
	Overview of My Year (New Year's Eve)	205
	Bibliotherapy: *Oh, The Places You'll Go* (Hot Air Balloons of Hope and The Places You'll Go Collage)	216